Praise for

HEAR & BEYOND

"In *Hear & Beyond*, Shari Eberts and Gael Hannan have created the ultimate survival guide to living well with hearing loss. For some readers, it will spark a sweeping life change. For others, it will be a turning point on their hearing loss journey. A must-read."

REBECCA ALEXANDER, LCSW-R, MPH, advocate; author, *Not Fade Away*

"This book is a game-changer! In *Hear & Beyond*, Gael Hannan and Shari Eberts offer a unique skills-based approach to living better with hearing loss. Its powerful strategies and engaging personal stories create a hopeful path forward for anyone affected by hearing loss."

BARBARA KELLEY, executive director, Hearing Loss Association of America

"Smart, funny, engaging. These three words sum up the easy-to-read and entirely enjoyable book *Hear & Beyond* by Gael Hannan and Shari Eberts. This duo are expert guides on living with hearing loss, and they do it with style. They give us specific strategies for communicating better, navigating romantic relationships, disclosing hearing loss in the workplace, and obtaining health care support, to cite a few examples. Most importantly, they share their mindset for meeting hearing challenges and encourage us to be our best selves. I highly recommend this book, for all—whether you have hearing loss or not, because, undoubtedly, you know someone who does."

RUTH WARICK, president, International Federation of Hard of Hearing People

"In *Hear & Beyond*, Shari Eberts and Gael Hannan provide a clear roadmap for individuals with hearing loss who want to hear and communicate better. There isn't a one-size-fits-all approach to communicating well with hearing loss, and *Hear & Beyond* provides the framework for individuals with hearing loss and their loved ones to know what to do."

FRANK LIN, MD, PhD, professor and director, Johns Hopkins Cochlear Center for Hearing and Public Health

"Gael Hannan and Shari Eberts bring two lifetimes of experience to their new book on hearing loss. *Hear & Beyond* is a valuable primer for those new to hearing loss and a reminder for those more experienced of the many skills, tools, and technologies available. Read this book start to finish or jump around as particular issues arise in your life. Gael and Shari may well have the key to helping you solve them."

KATHERINE BOUTON, former *New York Times* editor; author, *Smart Hearing*

"I've worn hearing aids since I was four years old, and I loved *Hear & Beyond*. It's full of empathy, experience, and real-world advice on navigating life as a person with hearing loss. This old, hard-of-hearing dog was very thankful to learn a few new tricks."

D.J. DEMERS, stand-up comedian with hearing loss

"*Hear & Beyond* is a must-read for people with hearing loss, their family members, and hearing health care professionals. As the authors state, there has been no operating manual for living a full and enriched life with hearing loss. Inspired by the lived experiences of authors Shari Eberts and Gael Hannan, this book comes as close to a 'hearing loss bible' as I have seen. Two thumbs up! A must-read for helping to unleash the full potential of people with hearing loss!"

BARBARA WEINSTEIN, founder, CUNY's Doctor of Audiology program

"This is a must-read for anyone who is using hearing devices, especially if you're new to this journey. I highly recommend this book! Shari Eberts and Gael Hannan went above and beyond to ensure you are empowered with tips and tricks for practically every situation."

DAWN HEIMAN, AuD, president-elect, Academy of Doctors of Audiology

"In *Hear & Beyond*, Shari Eberts and Gael Hannan have written the consumer hearing loss book that every hearing care professional should read. Their innovative yet practical model will benefit every person with hearing loss, their communication partners, and the professionals who serve them."

RICHARD SEEWALD, distinguished professor emeritus, National Centre for Audiology, Western University

"*Hear & Beyond* should be required reading for anyone living with hearing loss! Gael Hannan and Shari Eberts have written a hopeful and actionable guide for people to improve their abilities to communicate and live their best lives with hearing loss. Whether you have experienced hearing loss yourself or know someone who has, I cannot recommend *Hear & Beyond* enough!"

GLENN SCHWEITZER, tinnitus coach; author, *Rewiring Tinnitus* and *Mind Over Meniere's*

HEAR &
BEYOND

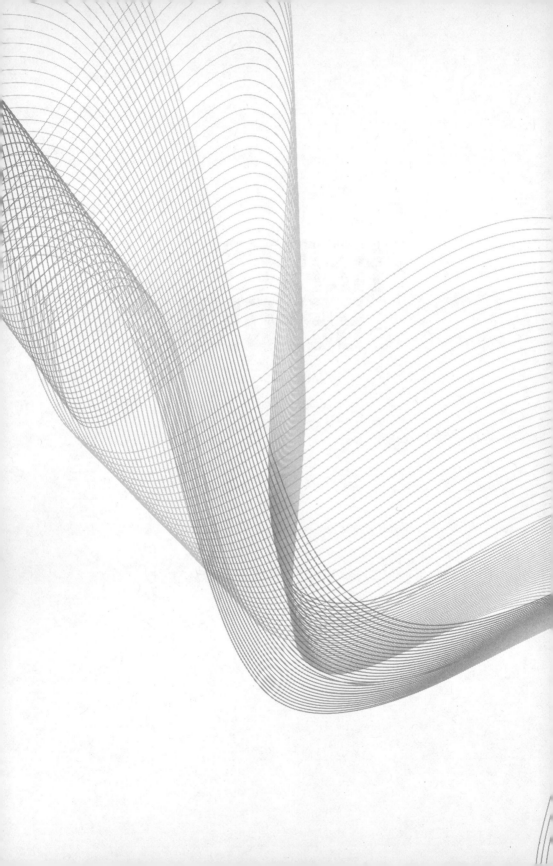

HEAR & BEYOND

Live Skillfully with Hearing Loss

SHARI EBERTS
GAEL HANNAN

PAGE TWO

Cataloguing in publication information is available from Library and Archives Canada.
ISBN 978-1-77458-160-5 (paperback)
ISBN 978-1-77458-161-2 (ebook)

Page Two
pagetwo.com

Edited by Kendra Ward
Copyedited by Rachel Ironstone
Proofread by Sara Harowitz
Cover and interior design by Jennifer Lum
Interior illustrations by Jeff Winocur
Printed and bound in Canada by Friesens
Distributed in Canada by Raincoast Books
Distributed in the US and internationally by Macmillan

22 23 24 25 26   5 4 3 2 1

HearAndBeyond.com
ShariEberts.com
GaelHannan.com

To all people living with hearing loss around the world.
You are not alone.

CONTENTS

RELATIONSHIPS AND SUPPORT NETWORKS:
Bringing Your People with You *161*

HEARING HACKS: Putting It All Together *223*

Introduction

THE ART OF LIVING SKILLFULLY WITH HEARING LOSS

WHAT IS IT like to live with hearing loss?
Those who have hearing loss find it hard to describe.
Those who don't have it find it hard to understand, especially in someone they love.

Why can you hear well in some situations but not in others? How can you be sensitive to loud noises, yet watch the TV at maximum volume? Why do the activities you once enjoyed now seem to take so much energy? Why don't hearing aids fix the problem the way glasses usually fix vision?

Whether you're new to hearing loss or have been living with it for a long time, you have probably felt the unwelcome change that hearing loss imposes on even the smallest corners of your communication life. With no operating manual to help you figure out

1

how to live with it, you've been getting by on information pieced together from various sources—yet communication often seems incomplete and unsatisfying.

You may be frustrated and isolated, perhaps even angry. These feelings are normal, shared at some point by almost everyone who has hearing loss—including your authors.

In our separate journeys, we struggled and found nothing changed, because we didn't know *how* to make things better. But eventually, through trial and error and the good fortune of meeting other amazing people with hearing loss, we each learned to live more skillfully. We shifted our focus from wanting to *hear* better to wanting to *communicate* better.

And that changed everything.

In *Hear & Beyond*, we offer a skills-based approach that will help you live better with your hearing loss, regardless of how long you've had it. Some strategies and workarounds will make a difference almost immediately, while others may take more time.

Our formula is based not only on our personal experiences but also on those of thousands of other people like us. Our principles are rooted in lived experiences and corroborated by hearing science, tremendous advances in technology, and the development of modern hearing care principles such as person-centered care.

In the chapters ahead, we share how our hard-won skills became personal philosophies for communication success. By simply opening yourself up to the *possibilities* of a new approach to your hearing loss, you're taking a transformational step forward.

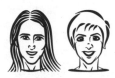

In our journeys,
we shifted our focus
from wanting to *hear*
better to wanting to
communicate better.

LIVING SKILLFULLY WITH HEARING LOSS

How *do* you live skillfully with hearing loss?

The first step is knowing what to expect. Understanding the big picture will help you embark on a more successful hearing loss journey.

The second key to living skillfully is introducing into your life a series of integrated strategies with a single, targeted purpose—to *improve communication*:

- changing your attitudes, which we call *MindShifts*;

- using a broad range of technology tools that boost comprehension; and

- changing the game with communication behaviors that make almost any listening situation manageable.

Think of this trio as the supports of a three-legged stool which never wobbles, even on bumpy ground. Each strategy is an important component of good communication, and when the three legs work together, they form a solid platform for your best possible communication life, supporting you in even the most challenging listening situations.

The final feature of skillful living is applying these strategies to the areas of life that matter most to you—in your relationships, work life, and other passions.

Hear & Beyond is structured around this simple framework:

- In "The Big Picture" we discuss the spectrum of experiences that comprise the hearing loss journey.

- In "MindShifts" we look at counter-productive attitudes and reframe them to help you live more successfully with hearing loss.

- In "Technology" we explore a variety of tools designed for better communication.

- In "Communication Game Changers" we reveal powerful non-technical strategies that can improve almost any difficult listening situation.

- In "Relationships and Support Networks" we describe how to build a strong and diverse support network, including choosing the right hearing care professional (HCP).

- In "Hearing Hacks" we offer specific tips for tackling everyday listening situations.

We have laid out the successful life with hearing loss as simply and clearly as we know how. No matter where you are on your hearing loss journey, it *can* be better if you want it to be. We know this because, like the millions of other people who live with hearing loss, we are on the journey with you.

What does it mean to live *skillfully* with hearing loss? Turn the page to find out.

THE BIG PICTURE
Understanding
the Journey

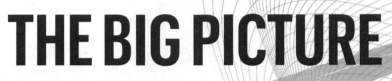

GAEL: For years, my life with hearing loss was a series of "I didn't know that" moments. I never knew what to expect, except that I would always have hearing loss because my doctor told me there would never be a cure in my lifetime. When I got my first hearing aid at age twenty, no one told me it would need replacing every five years or so. I didn't learn how to deal with the many emotions of hearing loss that affected my interactions with other people. I didn't know that I could do other things to improve communication, apart from lipreading, which happened almost naturally. I didn't have the big picture.

 SHARI: Exactly! Hearing loss isn't a one-time event—you get a hearing aid, and that's that. For most people, it's a continuous journey with stages that vary in duration and intensity, depending on a person's individual circumstances: type and degree of hearing loss; personality; attitudes; finances; levels of support from family, friends, and others; and so on.

 GAEL: No two journeys are exactly alike. The road to hearing loss success—however you define it—is straight for some people. For others, it's a meandering path with lots of doubling back and retracing steps. Straight or crooked, most paths have some detours along the way: fluctuations in hearing levels, life curveballs, or even new technology that needs getting used to all over again.

SHARI: The COVID-19 pandemic is a good example of that. Social distancing and masks rewrote the rules of effective communication. Even people who had been living comfortably for years with their hearing loss now struggled with the new challenges posed by trying to understand masked speech or to excel at video conferencing.

 GAEL: That's why the big picture is so important. If we understand what to expect from our hearing loss—such as the attitudes and emotions we may have about it, the technologies and non-technical tools we can use to communicate better, and how we can manage hearing loss in our relationships and our lives—then we can be prepared. We can manage our own journey.

 SHARI: If we knew then what we know now, the path would have had fewer bumps and less angst. The journey would have been easier, sooner.

1

THE JOURNEY
IS PERSONAL

HAT?

In a Wikipedia list of the hundred most-used English words, *what* ranks at number forty.[1] But for people with hearing loss who use the spoken word to communicate, the word *what* would probably crack the top ten list.

What? What did you say? What are we talking about? What did I miss?

What? is the perfect one-word description of life with hearing loss and its disconnect from free-flowing communication. Regardless of whether the loss is mild or profound, staying connected when you lose the thread of a discussion or miss a keyword is tough. Following a conversation takes a lot of effort—because you have to concentrate so hard to understand.

If you think you have hearing loss, you probably have some burning *what* questions of your own: *What do I do now? What happens next? What can I expect?*

If you have been living with hearing loss for a long time, perhaps for your entire life, you may feel frustrated or powerless: *What can I do to live better with my hearing loss, and who can help me?*

Unfortunately, hearing loss doesn't come with an operating manual. For decades, most hearing care professionals (HCPs) have followed a standard service model for clients whose hearing losses don't require medical intervention. They test and confirm a client's type and degree of hearing loss and create a treatment plan that usually involves hearing aid technology.

What's missing from this hearing care model is the big picture—a real-life illustration of how hearing loss, its emotions, and its barriers affect every corner of a person's life. The conventional approach ignores the many other strategies that a person needs in addition to hearing aids. Most HCPs don't paint this big picture for people with hearing loss, who are seldom invited to participate in developing their own go-forward plan for success.

We wish someone had told us there is more to living well with hearing loss than simply getting a hearing aid. It would have helped to realize sooner that hearing loss does not have to define us. We are not lesser-than or less deserving; hearing loss is only one aspect of who we are.

We have hearing loss, but it does not have us.

NO TWO JOURNEYS ARE ALIKE

No two people experience hearing loss in exactly the same way. We may pass through the same stages, but the route and timing of each phase will vary depending on personality, life circumstances, support networks, and ease of access to quality hearing care.

Your authors are the perfect example: Our stories share similarities, but also many differences. Gael's hearing loss began at birth, while Shari first noticed hers in her twenties; yet we both battled feelings of shame and stigma. Gael's parents and extended family were supportive while Shari's parents were less helpful. By today's standards, Gael should have started using assistive technology much earlier than age twenty, when she was finally prescribed a hearing aid. Shari's mild hearing loss allowed her to delay using hearing devices for many years.

Both of us developed robust support networks and built strong partnerships with our hearing care professionals. But not right away. While we managed careers, found supportive spouses, and raised children, we both experienced setbacks at various stages. We struggled with *tinnitus* (the experience of sound that has no external source) and battled fear and doubt. But we've been blessed with incredible advances in technology for traditional hearing aids and the proliferation of communication-boosting consumer devices and smartphone apps. Shari wears *bilateral hearing aids* (one in each ear). Gael is *bimodal*, meaning she wears a hearing aid in one ear and has a *cochlear implant* (a surgically implanted electronic hearing device) on the other side.

As you read our stories, you may find similarities to your own life. And you will also see that there is no formula for a perfect life with hearing loss. We, like you, continue to learn and to adapt to changes in our hearing and in our life, some of which are out of our control. Most importantly, in reading about our struggles and successes, you'll see that we are on this journey with you, urging you on to create your best life with hearing loss.

Shari: Battling Stigma, Embracing Change, Turning to Advocacy

Shari has an adult-onset genetic sensorineural bilateral progressive hearing loss. Sounds fancy, doesn't it? It means that her hearing loss was passed down through her family, although she first experienced symptoms as an adult. With *sensorineural* loss, the damage is not a structural flaw that can be repaired with surgery but an issue with the sensory cells or nerves. *Bilateral* refers to loss in both ears, and *progressive* means that, unfortunately, her hearing will likely continue to worsen over time.

She first noticed her hearing loss in her mid-twenties, when she was in graduate school, but her hearing loss journey began many years before, as she watched her father struggle with his own hearing challenges. He felt highly stigmatized by his hearing loss and did everything he could to hide it from everyone he knew, even growing his sideburns over his ears, long after it was fashionable, to hide his hearing aids. He eventually isolated himself from everyone, leading a lonely life until his passing several years ago.

At social gatherings, her father would disappear to a table in the corner, where he would sit by himself. Shari always wondered why he did this, but once her hearing loss began, she realized he probably couldn't hear well in the reverberant space, and was embarrassed or exhausted and just couldn't bring himself to bother trying to engage. Sadly, Shari's family was not supportive of him. Her mother often whispered to Shari and her sister behind their father's back, saying, "Don't worry, he can't hear us." Even as a child, Shari knew that wasn't nice, and thinking back on it now, she is horrified at the behavior. Perhaps her mother struggled with the stigma of hearing loss, too.

Shari's father's greatest fear was that somebody would discover his hearing loss, so he never asked anyone to speak louder or requested a quieter seat in a restaurant. He never did anything to draw attention to his hearing loss. Instead, he would often bluff, pretending to hear what others said rather than admit he had not.

Following in his footsteps, when Shari first began having hearing problems, she hid them. And when she got her first pair of hearing aids, she often refused to wear them, afraid that someone might see them. She was embarrassed, although she wasn't sure why. Was it a learned response from watching her father, or was it something larger—the societal stigma associated with hearing loss—that she wanted to avoid? In any event, her mother's reaction was not encouraging. "Do you really need to wear them?" she asked Shari.

Eventually, the answer became yes, Shari really did need to wear them, but still, she avoided them as much as possible. She would slip them in on the way to work, wearing them hidden behind long hair, and whip them back out as soon as the elevator door closed behind her on her way out of the office. When traveling, she would sneak them in before important client meetings. She hated her hearing aids and only wore them when she absolutely needed to, and never socially or with her family.

This all changed after she had children. Because her hearing loss is genetic, she feared she may have passed it on to them. She wanted to set a better example of how to thrive with hearing loss in case either of them should develop the condition. She started wearing her hearing aids all the time and learning about *assistive listening devices* (technologies other than hearing aids that improve communication in a variety of situations) and *hearing loops* (sound systems that transmit audio signals directly into a hearing aid via a magnetic field).

She taught her friends and family communication best practices and asked them to use them so she could hear her best. In 2014, she started *Living with Hearing Loss*, a blog and online community where she shares tips and tricks that she uses to live her best hearing loss life. She vowed that she would no longer allow her hearing loss to isolate her from the people that she loves or from the life that she wants to live. It takes effort, but it is worth it.

Now she is an advocate for people like her, writing and speaking about her life with hearing loss to raise awareness and improve communication access. Shari hopes that by sharing her story, she will help others live more comfortably with their own hearing issues.

Gael: Accepting, Adapting, Learning to Do Even Better

When someone asks Gael when she first became aware of her hearing loss, she always answers, "When my mommy told me."

Gael's mother was a nurse who realized that her two-year-old daughter was either very stubborn or had something else going on. The doctor confirmed *congenital hearing loss* (present at birth) of cause unknown. Was it her mother's challenging pregnancy or the even more difficult childbirth? Maybe it was because Gael was a tiny (and very cute) baby? Or perhaps it was related to some other health problem? There were no answers in her case.

Gael was always aware of her hearing issues—because she wasn't allowed to forget about them. At her annual trip to the pediatric ENT (ear, nose, and throat doctor, also referred to as an *otolaryngologist*), she was poked and prodded—up her nose and in her ears—and the verdict was always the same: "It's a little worse, come back next year. Sorry, a hearing aid won't help."

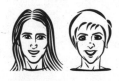

No two people experience hearing loss in exactly the same way.

She also couldn't ignore her hearing loss because her parents didn't. As she grew up, they emphasized the importance of good communication, encouraging her to speak clearly. *Slow down. Think about what you want to say. Let people know about your hearing loss.* Gael's teachers were always made aware, but the only educational strategy they could offer was for Gael to sit at the front of the class.

She was a good student, in spite of the lack of communication support—no hearing aids or other assistive devices and no teachers for students with hearing loss. It was not quite the dark age in terms of hearing loss, but almost. Although she didn't like sitting at the front all the time—her friends were usually at the back—it was her only hope of understanding her teachers, who had the annoying habit of turning their backs to write on the blackboard as they spoke. Only slightly better was their habit of walking around the classroom as they talked. She became a skilled rubbernecker because, as a speechreader (also known as a lipreader), her eyes followed the walking lips wherever they went.

The one time she decided to rebel and sit at the back of the class was a humiliating experience that haunts her still. The teacher called on her, but she hadn't heard clearly from the back. She stood up and, not wanting to say "pardon" in front of everyone, said, "Sorry, sir, I wasn't listening." Jaws dropped and the class went silent. The teacher said, "Well, thanks for sharing, Gael. But I was calling on Dale, not you." Next class, she was back at the front, having learned a basic hearing loss rule: Sit where you can see the lips.

At twenty, in a life-changing moment, she switched doctors and had a hearing aid within a month ... and life became really loud. Over the next two decades, as her hearing worsened, she depended on increasingly better hearing aids and useful strategies such as speechreading. She also used the common but not-so-beneficial tactic of bluffing her way through challenging listening situations.

Gael didn't *want* to have hearing loss. She felt inferior, although it would be years before she realized it. She was constantly embarrassed by her mishears, by saying the wrong things, for speaking too loudly, for cutting people off. She also tired of the constant struggle to understand and keep up with the conversation.

At forty, for the first time, she reached out to other people with hearing loss, a transformational decision that kickstarted a positive era in her journey. As she soaked up all the information she could about hearing loss—hers, anybody's, and everybody's—her negative attitudes faded away. She was stunned to learn that she was not alone and that for every communication challenge there are solutions. With this new outlook, she could allow other people to be her communication *partners*.

But living with hearing loss every day of your life doesn't necessarily mean you're good at it. On the contrary, people with hearing loss can become adept at ignoring their own needs, devising ways to hide their conditions and, worst of all, meekly putting up with inaccessible conditions simply because they don't know how to make it otherwise. To move forward, people with hearing loss must start by looking in the mirror and taking back control: *Okay, this is my life now. What am I going to do about it?*

Gael had this conversation with herself at forty, which spurred her to start using her talents to explain the hearing loss life. She created comedic-dramatic performances, became involved in advocacy projects, and presented across North America and internationally. She started writing, and in 2015 published her memoir and survival guide, *The Way I Hear It: A Life with Hearing Loss*. Life changed and her journey continues. Even now, the more she learns, the better she communicates.

2

THE FIVE STAGES
OF THE JOURNEY

ALTHOUGH EACH PERSON'S hearing loss journey is unique, the typical journey has five distinct stages. We've seen these in our personal experiences and in the lives of other people with hearing loss whom we have met through our decades-long work with consumer and professional hearing care organizations.

The length of each stage is determined by individual circumstances and how each person deals with them. Some people never move beyond the first stage, choosing to live in denial of their hearing loss. Other people get a hearing aid and think they've done all they need to do to hear better.

But that doesn't have to be you! When you understand the big picture and what to expect from the hearing loss journey, you will recognize the power you have to create the life you want.

Stage 1: Debating with yourself. You wonder if you're having trouble hearing or if everyone else is mumbling. These suspicions may be subconscious as you struggle with denial, looking for anything or anyone else to blame but your own poor hearing.

Stage 2: Validating. It's official. In a series of evaluations, your HCP confirms that you have a hearing loss. It may not be what you wanted, but it's now a reality.

Stage 3: Taking charge. With your hearing loss confirmed, you decide to do something about it. Depending on the type of loss, hearing aids are often the first step, but you may discover they are not a stand-alone prescription for hearing loss. Other changes need to be made. You learn as much as you can about your hearing loss and begin to adopt a dynamic and interlacing set of mental, technical, and practical communication strategies.

Stage 4: Living skillfully. This phase is the ultimate goal for your life with hearing loss. In your daily activities and your relationships, you apply what you learned when you took charge in Stage 3. You are open-minded about adopting new strategies and technologies that can improve your daily communications.

Stage 5: Refreshing and restarting. Just when you think you have it all figured out, something changes. This is what makes the hearing loss experience an ongoing journey rather than a puzzle with a finite solution. Hearing aids need replacing, hearing levels might change, or some other event comes along to change the rules of engagement. Any of these may reroute you to a previous point in your journey. It's a natural part of the process and an opportunity to try something new and to become even more skillful.

The stages described here don't happen overnight. They can happen quickly, over the course of a few months, but are more likely to stretch over years. You may need more time to assess your own situation and abilities. You may require time to build your resolve and confidence so that you can try something new. Give yourself the space to ask questions, of others and of yourself.

Achieving hearing success is not a time-limited offer. There are no hard start or stop dates. Some people wait years before finally deciding to do something about their hearing loss. Others just snap to it and race off down the road.

For most of us, the journey with hearing loss will last a lifetime. Take a look at the big picture and make it yours—and the sooner the better, because there's a world of improved communication waiting for you.

Let's take a deeper dive into what happens in each stage.

STAGE 1: DEBATING WITH YOURSELF

"What did he say?" Shari whispered to her seatmate in class. The room had just exploded in laughter at something the teacher said. This wasn't the first time Shari had missed a punchline. Early into her first semester of graduate school, she began worrying about her hearing. She started missing comments that students made under their breath and the quiet jokes that set the room ablaze with laughter. She knew what was happening. She was losing her hearing, just like her father had as a young adult.

If you are genetically predisposed to hearing issues, it may be easier to recognize them in yourself. But for most people there is no single *aha* moment when they finally realize or admit to a problem. Hearing loss often develops so gradually it may be hard to notice in yourself. Most often a family member notices it first, perhaps during the nightly battle over the volume of the television or because of the innocent comment that was misinterpreted as anger. Socializing is no longer as enjoyable; in fact, it is exhausting.

For most people, this stage, marked with feelings of denial, fear, and anger, lasts the longest: an average of seven to ten years!

Signs of Hearing Loss

Acknowledging that you may have hearing loss is the first big step towards better hearing. The signs are all there—you just need to recognize them:

You frequently say "What?" This is the stereotypical sign of someone with a hearing problem, but that doesn't make it any less true. If you ask people to repeat themselves frequently, the issue is probably with you, not them.

You hear people talk but do not understand what they say. This is the biggest giveaway. You hear the sound of a voice, but you don't understand what is being said. Blaming this on a mumbling conversation partner is all too easy, but when it occurs frequently, and in quiet surroundings, it is a strong indicator of hearing problems.

You set the TV volume too loud for others. This is one of the most obvious signs of hearing loss, and one that only others will recognize.

Talking with people exhausts you. When you have hearing loss, hearing is no longer something that happens automatically in the background while you handle other tasks. It is an activity that requires effort. This extra concentration can be exhausting, especially if your day is filled with lots of socializing or group meetings.

You avoid socializing or talking on the phone. This is the greatest risk of untreated hearing loss—social withdrawal and isolation. Over time it can lead to depression as well as cognitive problems, such as a higher risk of developing dementia. If you notice that you are making excuses not to do the things you used to love, hearing loss may be at least part of the reason.

You secretly lipread. If it bothers you when people cover their mouths while speaking to you or when their back is turned, you're probably depending on speechreading cues like lip movements and facial expressions to help you hear. People with typical hearing do this, too, but if you rely on it in a conversation, you are probably not hearing as well as you should be.

You hear better at home than when out and about. Background noise makes it harder for people with hearing loss to understand speech. If it is much easier for you to hear at home or in a quiet office than it is to hear in a coffee shop, restaurant, or shopping mall, hearing loss may be the reason.

The Inner Wrestling Begins

At the first suggestion of hearing loss, the inner debate begins. You may battle shame and embarrassment or suffer feelings of loss. You may weigh the pros and cons of acknowledging your hearing problems. *I do fine most of the time, why bother?* This internal debate is normal, and it is an important step in ultimately accepting your hearing loss.

You may be experiencing:

Denial: Why is everyone mumbling? If they turned down the background music, I could hear my dinner companions just fine.

Grief can happen at any stage. When I received my cochlear implant, I wept for all the wonderful new sounds that I had been missing until then.

Fear: What if it's true? How will my life change? Can I function at my job? As a parent? As a spouse? Will I face discrimination?

Anger: Why can't people speak more clearly? Why is my spouse such a low talker? Why can't my boss keep her hands away from her mouth when she talks to me? This is not fair.

Shame: How will society view me? Why are people with hearing loss often the brunt of the joke? Will I appear stupid or slow? Will my friends and loved ones accept me?

Sadness: I feel isolated from family and friends. I don't want to socialize anymore because I can't hear what people are saying. Nobody works to include me in the conversation. I missed the punchline of the joke again. I am unhappy.

It's Okay to Mourn

Some people have experienced hearing loss their entire lives. It's their reality and they may or may not be comfortable with it. Others take pride in their deafness and don't feel they have lost anything. But for many, regardless of how long they have lived with it, hearing loss is just that—a loss that has affected their ability to function easily in society, to connect with loved ones, and to enjoy intimate moments and entertainment. It is a loss of freedom, of confidence, and even of feelings of self-worth. It can be devastating, especially if you are also plagued by feelings of stigma, fearing others will view you negatively because of your hearing loss.

Allow yourself to grieve.

You may also feel guilty about how your hearing loss impacts your loved ones. And, in turn, your family's attitudes about your hearing loss may influence your outlook. For example, parents may be in denial and encourage their hard of hearing child not to talk about the "problem" and to keep hearing aids hidden. You may feel that your spouse is embarrassed by your hearing loss, or regret that you must depend on your child to interpret for you by repeating what someone else just said.

Your desire to wallow in self-pity and guilt is understandable, but don't make this your permanent state. Take the next step. This means having an HCP evaluate your hearing and validate your concerns.

STAGE 2: VALIDATING

You may spend seven to ten years, give or take, arriving at this moment. But once you admit to yourself that you likely have hearing loss, it is time to confirm it.

Different types of professionals may be involved. You might be referred to an ear, nose, and throat (ENT) doctor for an initial diagnosis and to rule out or deal with other medical conditions of the hearing system. If you are having difficulty hearing and it is not sudden in onset, you may prefer to go to an audiologist or hearing instrument specialist. The difference between the two lies in their training and professional scope.

Audiologists are regulated health care professionals, usually with master's degrees or doctorates, who evaluate and manage hearing loss and other hearing-related disorders. *Hearing instrument specialists* are professionals specifically trained to test hearing and dispense hearing aids. In this book, we use the general term hearing care professional (HCP) to refer to either of these trained clinicians who evaluate a possible hearing loss and offer a course of treatment.

A full evaluation includes a physical examination of your ears, several types of hearing tests, and a consultation with an HCP. Consider bringing a family member with you to provide moral support and a second set of ears for the HCP's recommendations. Family members can also provide valuable input about the types of hearing situations that are most challenging for you. The entire process is painless and usually takes sixty to ninety minutes.

Your First Hearing Assessment

The first appointment can feel scary. Even arranging the initial appointment can be challenging if you have trouble hearing on the phone. You wonder if you have found the right HCP, what will happen when you are there, and what, if anything, you will learn. These are common feelings, but try to approach the appointment with an open mind. Your HCP is a true partner in helping you hear and communicate better—assuming you can find one that practices person-centered care. We discuss this in greater detail in Chapter 26.

In your first consultation, the HCP should ask you about the types of communication difficulties you are having. The more specific you are in your answers the better. Prepare before the appointment by listing the listening situations you find difficult and the most important activities for which you need hearing assistance. This will focus the conversation on what is most important to you and your lifestyle.

In the physical exam, the HCP examines your ears for anything that might be blocking the sound from reaching the inner ear. This could be a buildup of wax, other physical obstructions, or a deformity of the bones of the middle ear. Hearing loss caused by a blockage or physical defect in the outer or middle part of the ear is called a *conductive hearing loss* and may be reversible with medical treatment. However, most hearing loss is *sensorineural,* caused by damage to the inner ear sensory cells or because of problems with the nerve connection between the ear and the brain. Sensorineural hearing loss is often permanent, with some exceptions.

The physical exam is followed by a series of hearing tests in a sound booth. The process might vary slightly among clinics, but you will wear headphones and respond to a series of tones at different frequencies in each ear. When you hear the tone, you press the buzzer. This test is then repeated without the headset, with a small square-like black box placed behind your ear instead. The test results are compared to determine the type of hearing loss.

The final evaluations test your ability to understand the spoken word. The HCP sets the volume to a comfortable level and asks you to repeat a series of words. One test uses monosyllabic words such as *keep* and *this* to assess word recognition, while another tests sound sensitivity using familiar compound words such as *baseball* and *hot dog*. You might leave the sound booth hungry and ready for a day at the ballpark. Or your head might be resonating with all the sounds you've heard.

Shari has always been an eager test-taker—it is just in her DNA to try to do well on tests. Perhaps that makes her a bit overzealous and explains why she tends to have many false positives in her hearing tests. When she reviews the results, she sometimes wonders if the stability reflected in the test is real or if she just got lucky with her impassioned button pressing.

Gael has never looked forward to hearing tests—mainly because not once in her decades of hearing evaluations has an HCP said, "Well done, Gael! Your hearing has improved!" She often feels anxious before a test, especially if she suspects that her hearing has dropped a bit or a lot. She believes hearing professionals should find ways to encourage their clients to relax before the evaluation. (Wine might help.)

In truth, you can't fail a hearing test. Struggling to hear the words or being unsure whether you heard a beep may feel like a failure, but these tests are not about winning or losing. They establish whether you have hearing loss and, if you do, the type and degree of loss.

Once the testing is complete, your HCP will explain the results and share recommendations. You will receive your *audiogram*, a pictorial representation of your hearing that shows how loud tones of different frequencies need to be for you to hear them. The x-axis displays the frequency or pitch of the sound measured in hertz (Hz), and the y-axis shows the necessary loudness of each tone measured in decibels (dB). The slope of the line provides useful information about the severity of your loss across the spectrum of frequencies.

For example, age-related hearing loss typically occurs in the high frequencies, meaning sounds like birds' chirps, doorbells, and young children's voices are often the hardest to hear. Many important speech sounds, like *s*, *th*, and *f*, also occur in these high frequencies. Your audiogram will help you understand which sounds and voices are most difficult for you to hear. Ask to see the *speech banana*, which is a simplified illustration of where the speech sounds fall on the scale of frequency (pitch) and loudness. A person's audiogram is overlaid on the chart to show the parts of spoken language that are likely hardest for them to understand without assistance.

Based on your audiogram, your HCP will determine the degree and type of your hearing loss and your particular hearing and sound-processing needs. Hearing loss is often described as *mild*, *moderate*, *severe*, or *profound*, with several gradations between. But this standard scale may be overly simplistic because the categories don't indicate how well a person functions. For example, a person with severe hearing loss may cope better than another person who is assessed with moderate loss because of differences in their personality, life situation, and attitudes—for example, their willingness to advocate for their hearing needs. Similarly, a person with normal hearing as measured on the audiogram may have difficulty communicating with others for the same reasons. Don't attach too much importance to your assigned category; it's your ability to communicate, not the label, that is the key.

If your hearing loss is conductive, you will be referred to an ENT for further examination. However, the most common type of hearing loss is sensorineural, and with one or two exceptions, the standard treatment option is technology. For most people this means traditional hearing aids, but not always. For people with mild to moderate hearing loss, direct-to-consumer hearing devices known as *hearables* may be a good first step.

People with severe and profound hearing loss and people for whom hearing aids are no longer helpful may be candidates for a cochlear implant, a surgically implanted device that bypasses the sensory cells in the inner part of the ear and generates electrical signals to stimulate the auditory nerve and send the message to the brain for processing. We discuss various technology options in Chapters 7 to 11.

Hearing Is Critical to Your Overall Health

Even when your test results indicate hearing loss, you may still have mixed feelings about getting hearing aids. You may revisit the same feelings of stigma, denial, and fear you wrestled with before. This is a natural response, and it may take some time before you are ready to take the hearing aid plunge.

But eventually you must stop thinking about it and do it. Hearing health is a critical part of your overall well-being, and although it may be tempting to ignore your hearing loss, especially if you can "make it work" most of the time, this is unwise.

In addition to the social isolation, sadness, and frustration that often come with untreated hearing loss, there are many medical reasons to take care of your hearing. Hearing loss is associated with several serious health issues, including diabetes and cardiovascular disease.[2] It is correlated with a higher risk of falls.[3] Many cases of tinnitus (internal ringing or other sounds in the ears) also occur in conjunction with hearing loss.

Studies also show a higher risk of dementia in people with untreated hearing loss. A 2011 study conducted by Frank Lin, the director of the Cochlear Center for Hearing and Public Health at Johns Hopkins Bloomberg School of Public Health, showed that even people with mild hearing loss were twice as likely to develop dementia than those with normal hearing, and that this likelihood increased with higher degrees of hearing loss.[4] More research is being done to determine why this occurs.

But—don't panic! Having hearing loss does not mean you will develop dementia. The study refers to people with *untreated* hearing loss, and subsequent studies show that wearing hearing devices may lower or forestall the risk of cognitive decline.[5] Researchers are looking into whether one condition causes the other or if they are both related to a separate underlying condition. Whatever they discover, the important and clear message is that your hearing health is critical to your ability to remain socially connected and to your overall well-being in more ways than just hearing. Don't ignore it.

STAGE 3: TAKING CHARGE

You have acknowledged your hearing loss, have gathered professional validation and advice, are dealing with the insecurities and emotions, and have decided to improve your life. You are entering the most transformational part of your hearing loss journey.

Taking control of your hearing loss involves three fundamental strategies:

- changing your attitudes, which we call MindShifts;

- using a broad range of technology tools that boost comprehension; and

- changing the game with communication behaviors that make almost any listening situation manageable.

In the introduction, we referred to these strategies as the three legs of a stool. We encourage you to embrace all three because, together, they create a strong and stable platform for skillful living with hearing loss. Each of these crucial strategies is the focus of the next three parts of this book.

Of the three major groups of skills, MindShifts may be the most important. People with hearing loss can adopt technology and use the best communication practices, but without a can-do attitude towards hearing loss, the other strategies simply will not work as well. Put another way, an optimistic attitude will make your hearing aids work better and your conversations more engaging!

Using these strategies together, though, brings the magic to skillful living with hearing loss. Even after Shari accepted her hearing loss and began wearing hearing aids all the time, there were still many situations when she felt lost. It took years to build her bag of hearing tricks and technologies and to develop the right mindset to advocate for herself. Once she did, things got much easier.

STAGE 4: LIVING SKILLFULLY

And then you've done it! You have devices you trust, you use communication best practices, and you advocate for your needs. You regularly apply these strategies in your communications and have developed the confidence to take on almost any new hearing loss challenge. Most of the time. Or maybe just some of the time.

Gael allows herself one "Bad Hearing Day" a year. On this day, in her head or alone somewhere, it's okay to get mad at people for mumbling, to be furious at a husband who once again forgot the rules, and to become incensed at her own bluffing or neglect in advocating for her needs. She can cry when she can't hear what everyone else hears. She can cringe with embarrassment at her verbal boo-boos when she doesn't hear something correctly. This annual rant achieves absolutely nothing except to give in to the relief of ranting. The next day she's back at it, hearing as hard as she can, moving forward.

There are rough moments and bad days when your hearing seems to have dropped through the floor and all your hard-earned skills seem to fail you. But these moments pass, and soon you are back to living skillfully with your hearing loss.

STAGE 5: REFRESHING AND RESTARTING

Just when your life with hearing loss seems to be relatively smooth sailing, something changes. Your hearing does a small nosedive. Your HCP retires. You need new hearing aids. Your overall health changes. Maybe a global crisis delivers a new set of communication challenges or perhaps life events have spurred a new bout of anxiety or other emotion.

If there's one thing we know for sure in life is that *stuff happens*. And when it affects our life with hearing loss, we need to make changes. We may need to double back to a previous stage.

Think of this phase of the journey as the shoulder of the highway. It allows you to pull over and turn around if you need to, for whatever reason. Maybe you want to rest just for a bit, to calm down after a stressful listening situation, or you want to figure out how to deal with a relationship that is strained by your hearing loss. You may need to consider new technology or whether to get a cochlear implant, or simply pause to think about where you want to go next.

Then, when you're ready, you can pull back onto the road to wherever you're headed. This shoulder is always there for you, and you *will* use it from time to time. It's part of living a normal life with hearing loss.

Note: Whatever stage of the journey you are in, if your hearing drops suddenly and drastically, this is a medical emergency. Immediately contact your HCP and head to the emergency room.

3

WHEN YOU ALSO EXPERIENCE TINNITUS

A S IF HEARING loss were not enough to deal with on its own, sometimes it comes with related hearing and balance problems. The most common of these is tinnitus, which is the internal perception of sound that has no external source. Tinnitus should not be ignored. It is usually caused by an underlying condition, such as hearing loss, an ear injury, or a problem with the circulatory system, although it is often difficult to determine the cause.

Tinnitus sufferers report hearing sounds that range from a persistent ringing bell to a cacophony of different noises with more than a hundred variations in between. It may pulse along with your heartbeat or be triggered by repetitive noises. Regardless of how it sounds to a person, the impact of tinnitus can be mild to extremely debilitating. According to the British Tinnitus Association, about 30 percent of people will experience tinnitus at some point in their lives.[6]

Shari's tinnitus is most often a high-pitched ring, while Gael's head noise is harder to describe. Imagine a badly led orchestra where musicians play their own music on their own beat, creating a painful discordance of hums, thumps, clanging, shrieking, and ghostly whooshing.

Gael also has *hyperacusis*—an extreme sensitivity to ordinary environmental sounds—which is far less common than tinnitus, although the two often coexist. What someone who experiences hyperacusis may hear as painfully loud is perceived at normal levels by another person. The sensation of loudness may come and go or be constant. For many, the condition is extremely debilitating.

Vertigo is a specific kind of dizziness where a person experiences the sensation that they are spinning or the room is spinning. It can have many causes, some of which are related to hearing loss, such as Meniere's disease.

If you experience tinnitus, hyperacusis, or vertigo, talk to your doctor.

TREATMENT OPTIONS FOR TINNITUS

For some people, tinnitus is loud enough to overpower other sounds, even speech sounds, making conversation difficult. For others, the perceived sound can be masked by wearing hearing aids or by playing soft music. People who suffer from its relentless presence will usually try anything to get rid of it.

There is not yet a cure for tinnitus, making it a challenging disorder for physicians and HCPs to treat. When you ask your doctor for help you may be told, "Sorry, there's nothing we can do. Just get used to it." Do not accept this response.

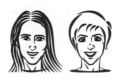

We share a passionate belief in the power of meditation and yoga to lessen the intensity and emotional impact of tinnitus.

There *are* ways to make living with tinnitus easier. Because tinnitus is an individual experience—in what it sounds like and how it affects us emotionally—the methods we use to alleviate our symptoms are also different. For example, dietary changes like reducing salt, alcohol, and caffeine are helpful for some people but not others. Getting enough rest or sleep and sufficient hydration will help almost everyone, but beware of advertised quick fixes like specific vitamins, special compounds, or food combinations. Usually these "cures" are nothing more than a waste of time and money.

Masking to Reduce the Sound

To deal with the relentless sounds of your tinnitus, try masking them with other sounds.

Wearing hearing aids provides relief for some people because it increases the volume of ambient noise. This works for Shari and is one of the reasons she uses extended-wear hearing aids. Certain hearing aids also come with a tinnitus setting that can be programmed to offset the specific tone of your tinnitus. Other ways to mask tinnitus include using white noise machines, playing music in the background, or keeping a TV on at a low volume.

Meditation, Focus Shifts, and Exercise

Tinnitus has a terrifying power to occupy not only our heads but our thoughts, driving up our stress and immobilizing us. But our brains offer us a wonderful gift—the ability to stop feeling unpleasant things by focusing on something more pleasant. Whether it's watching a good show, reading, or talking with friends, when you allow yourself to be drawn into the enjoyment of these activities, you can, if even just for a little while, stop "hearing" your head noise. This may not be easy to do in the early days or months of tinnitus, but when you learn to give other things more importance than your tinnitus, you weaken its ability to affect you.

We are passionate believers in the power of meditation, yoga, and deep, intentional breathing to lessen the intensity and emotional impact of tinnitus. Shari discovered meditation almost by accident at a yoga retreat many years ago. The impact was almost immediate. When she sat quietly and focused on her breathing during the meditations, her tinnitus eased into the background. After many months and years of regular meditation, her tinnitus is thankfully well controlled for most of the year, with one exception—when the weather turns cold each winter.

Gael, however, could deep breathe for hours on end and her tinnitus would still be there. She is, nonetheless, a convert to the power of short meditations and deep, intentional breathing. They calm her and allow her to shift her focus to a better place—which is anywhere but her tinnitus.

Meditating can be simple. Sit quietly for ten minutes, and you've done it. If that sounds too hard, use an app that offers guided meditations that walk you through the steps. Or just take some deep breaths—in through the nose and out through the mouth. Even if it doesn't help with tinnitus, it may still be time well spent and a brief antidote to the stress of daily life.

Physical exercise also has a positive impact on tinnitus. When the body has a robust workout, it releases endorphins that diminish the perception of pain. Exercise is also a powerful stress reliever which allows you to function better, even in the presence of irritating head noise. Consider adding daily exercise to your tinnitus-be-gone plan.

Cognitive Behavioral Therapy

Cognitive behavioral therapy (CBT) uses techniques including relaxation, discussion, and problem-solving skills to change the way a person responds to negative stimuli. When successful, it retrains your emotional response to tinnitus, making it more manageable. The tinnitus does not go away, but your response to it changes for the better.

CBT is most often conducted one-on-one with a trained professional, but there are also apps available to fill in when individual counseling is not possible.

Peer Support

Finding others who share your experiences with tinnitus can be a huge help. Not only will others commiserate with you, but they may also have suggestions for easing the strain. Talking about the problem and sharing stories is therapeutic. There are many social media groups and online forums for people with tinnitus. Your HCP may also refer you to a professional tinnitus management course.

Like hearing loss itself, there is no complete medical cure currently available for tinnitus. Treatments lie in finding ways to manage tinnitus to reduce its impact and frequency. If you have tinnitus (or hyperacusis or vertigo), we encourage you to seek professional guidance as well as peer support.

MINDSHIFTS
A New Approach to Hearing Loss

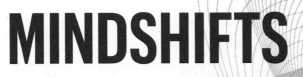

SHARI: When Gael and I started working on this book, we spent a lot of time discussing the strategies that can make the hearing loss life "livable." We quickly discovered that both of us—at some point in our individual journeys and in different ways—experienced a startling shift in how we thought and what we believed about our hearing loss.

 GAEL: Our attitudes towards our hearing loss had changed, and suddenly the hearing loss itself changed! I couldn't hear any better than I did before, but how I operated as a person with hearing loss was better. Less stress, more confidence, more success.

 SHARI: Me too—better attitudes turned into better conversations because I was more positive. I stopped viewing my hearing loss as an enemy that I always had to fight because it made me "lesser than" other people.

 GAEL: Although calling it a friend that we love might be going too far. How about a companion that we accept— because it's not going to leave! Like you, Shari, I just stopped thinking of myself as diminished and realized that I deserved to hear and be heard. The transformation was a lightbulb moment that I still remember with a tingle.

 SHARI: Mine was a longer process but just as life chang- ing. It was a triumph of attitude change—what we call a MindShift.

4

CHANGING YOUR MIND

A HEARING LOSS DIAGNOSIS often comes with emotional burdens that paint hearing loss as embarrassing or shameful or, at the very least, something never to be discussed. Some of these beliefs come from external sources like advertisements, TV shows, and other media that use poor hearing as the brunt of jokes or to make someone appear stupid or out of touch. Without realizing it, we often internalize these feelings, looking down on ourselves, causing us to hide our hearing loss so that we don't appear weak or broken:

This must be a mistake! I'm too young for hearing loss!

People will think I'm old or incompetent.

I do not want hearing loss or hearing aids! Maybe it's wax?

My friend with hearing aids says they don't even work—and they cost so much!

Why is everyone mumbling?

If any of these thoughts has gone through your mind, you're not alone. Most of us have an unpleasant gut reaction to the enormous change caused by hearing loss. We want what we once took for granted—easy interactions with people, confidence on the job, and effortless enjoyment of music, television, and personal devices. With hearing loss, our self-perception may also change, shifting from viewing ourselves as someone capable to someone who is "lesser than." We experience self-doubt. We may feel broken or weak. We have internalized the negative societal attitudes about hearing loss and made them our own, and while these attitudes are false, they seem real to *us*, and we feel their weight.

But we may not be aware of the stress and negative emotions we are carrying. Anger, fear, and resentment might be simmering just below our consciousness. Even if we use hearing aids, the psychological turmoil can persist, and when allowed to fester, these stresses can lead to depression and social isolation. They prevent us from moving forward and living skillfully with our hearing loss.

Consider this: *Our attitudes towards hearing loss affect our emotions and behaviors.* This is a powerful statement. It means life with hearing loss can be different—perhaps better than you thought—just by changing your attitudes. If you can reframe your unproductive, destructive thoughts by pulling them out of their hard place and repositioning them as constructive, *actionable* statements, you create a healthier approach to hearing loss. We call this process a MindShift.

Behavioral change doesn't happen overnight; attitudes— entrenched ways of thinking that guide feelings and behavior—can be sticky. Many of the negative societal attitudes, often based on misunderstandings about deafness, have existed for centuries.

"Mild hearing loss" is a bit of a misnomer. If you can't communicate well with others, this is not a *mild* problem—it is a serious one.

Even slight improvements in your thinking can positively affect your behavior. When you transform barriers into stepping-stones to success, you are experiencing MindShifts.

WHY ARE MINDSHIFTS IMPORTANT?

MindShifts are not "cures" for hearing loss. You can't heal your hearing loss through vitamin therapy, cochlear massages, or breathing in peppermint fumes. And—reality check—even the best hearing aid in the world won't "fix" hearing loss, because science and medicine are just not there yet. But when you actively support your hearing aids with other strategies, including an improved emotional attitude, you *can* communicate better.

We are not trying to over-simplify or minimize the impact of hearing loss on your life. Even mild hearing loss can cause problems with communication—and communication is the glue that connects us to each other. Hearing loss tears away at this glue, causing problems in relationships, work, and self-esteem.

It's worth repeating that your goal should be to communicate better, not simply to hear better. If hearing better is all that you're aiming for, aim higher. Technology has its limits. Better communication doesn't.

TAKE AN ATTITUDE SELFIE!

Wouldn't it be nice if you could simply look at a list of negative attitudes, check off the ones you think you have, say "be gone!" and, poof, they disappear?

Thinking back, Gael realized that she blamed her hearing loss for many things that weren't quite right in her life. Relationships, lack of assertiveness, being left out of things. She knew she didn't like being "hard of hearing" but she didn't realize the depth of her stress until she witnessed what a more proactive attitude towards hearing loss could produce. She had been operating under a negative set of life rules and suddenly understood that having hearing loss is okay—that it is, in fact, normal. Technology became her friend. With these thoughts, she walked taller and probably smiled more.

How do you improve your attitude? You can begin by acknowledging that you are responsible for managing your own hearing problems. Stop looking *outward* for places to lay the blame for poor communication in your life. You didn't cause your hearing loss, but only *you* can improve your communication.

Start by taking a snapshot of your attitudes towards hearing loss.

When we take selfies with our cameras or phones, we are often surprised at what we see. "I don't look like that, do I?" Your attitude selfie might surprise you. Perhaps you hold yourself to a double standard; you accept hearing loss in other people but not in yourself. You may discover other attitudes that are blocking you from better communication.

Take this attitude selfie. Read the following statements to see if they describe how you feel about your hearing loss:

- Why me?

- Nobody understands what I'm going through.

- I want to hear better, the way I used to.

- I don't like to advertise my hearing loss. People will think I'm old or slow.

- My family and friends always forget about my hearing loss.

- Hearing aids are ugly, expensive, and don't always work.

- I don't want to bother anybody with my hearing loss needs.

- Who would want to hire me? Or love me? Or be my friend?

- I get angry at myself and others when we make communication mistakes.

- Everywhere I go, there is no access for people with hearing loss.

What did you find? Did you recognize any, some, or all of these attitudes as yours?

Do I really think like that? Maybe I do.

Time for a MindShift.

5

THE MINDSHIFTS

LET'S TAKE ANOTHER look at that list of unproductive mindsets—some of which you may recognize in yourself. This time, each attitude is reframed as an *actionable* statement. Each transition is a powerful MindShift.

Attitude	The MindShift
Why me?	I have the potential to change my journey. The person with the most power in my hearing loss success is *me*.
Nobody understands what I'm going through.	Many people experience the same challenges as I do. I can learn from them. I'm not alone.
I want to hear better, the way I used to.	I want to *communicate* better, and it takes more than hearing aids to do this. I must use other skills and additional technology.
I don't like to advertise my hearing loss. People will think I'm old or slow.	Being open about my hearing loss will help me communicate better. Trying to hide my hearing loss leads to misunderstandings.

Attitude	The MindShift
My family and friends always forget about my hearing loss.	My hearing loss impacts my family and friends, too. We will learn how to be better communicators together.
Hearing aids are ugly, expensive, and don't always work.	Technology is my friend. My devices let me hear sounds I had forgotten or had never heard before. They connect me to other people and the world.
I don't want to bother anybody with my hearing loss needs.	I deserve to hear and be heard. I deserve to participate.
Who would want to hire me? Or love me? Or be my friend?	Hearing loss is just one aspect of who I am. I'm comfortable with myself. I have skills, smarts, and love to share.
I get angry at myself and others when we make communication mistakes.	Communication improves with practice. I forgive myself when I'm not perfect. I am grateful for the efforts of others, even when they're not perfect.
Everywhere I go, there is no access for people with hearing loss.	It is my right to ask for and receive equal access. When I advocate for myself, I am also creating change that benefits others.

What follows in this chapter is a closer look at three of these Mind-Shifts to demonstrate the powerful impact of adopting a new approach to your hearing loss.

WHY ME?

As a teenager with hearing loss, Gael wondered "Why me?" Her friends didn't need to sit at the front of the class in school. They could whisper and share secrets. She felt left out. Over time—a long time, actually—she realized that there often isn't a good answer to that question, except "Why *not* you?"

The human body is amazing, but it is organic and therefore prone to breakdown. As an adult, Gael gained a better perspective: Everybody has to deal with some health or social issue. Some people get more than their share of bad luck, and their cries of "Why me?" are far more loaded with suffering. So, if she catches herself feeling like a victim, she reminds herself that she has options and she is the only one who can take advantage of them.

"Why me?" can be a tough question to answer, and partly because the question can mean two different things.

You might mean "How did I get this hearing loss, what caused it?" Not everyone can find the answer to this question because there are many causes of hearing loss. It could be hereditary, running in the family for generations. It could also be because of birth issues: low birthweight, maternal health, even a traumatic birth process. Childhood ear infections are a common culprit. Hearing loss can be caused by trauma to the head or ear, or an acoustical trauma resulting in noise-induced hearing loss. Poor listening habits—too loud for too long over time—can result in permanent hearing loss. Sometimes hearing loss occurs suddenly without any apparent explanation—in many cases of hearing loss, the cause remains unknown.

Perhaps, though, your question is one of despair, of feeling victimized. Of all the weights you could carry, couldn't you have pulled the short straw for something else? You might think, *No one, no one, has got it as bad as I do! Hearing loss touches every single corner of my life, and* nothing *fixes it!*

It's a hard place to be, engulfed in this feeling of helplessness. But the pain can become the impetus for change, as hard as it might seem. In the simple act of reading this book, you are moving forward.

Our lives are different because we have hearing loss, but maybe that's not a totally bad thing. Shari's life is now full of wonderful people that she would not have met if it weren't for her hearing issues; people who understand her and who have helped her become an advocate for equal access. She believes she's become a better mother and a better life partner since she changed her perspective about her hearing loss.

> **MindShift**
> I have the potential to change my journey. The person with the most power in my hearing loss success is *me*.

NOBODY UNDERSTANDS WHAT I'M GOING THROUGH

When Shari was diagnosed with hearing loss in her mid-twenties, she didn't know anybody with hearing loss other than her father. But he wasn't going to talk about it with her. He was already beaten down by the stigma and shame he felt about his hearing issues. She felt alone and misunderstood. Sometimes she could hear well, other times she couldn't. She didn't feel comfortable asking for help, and even if she had, she didn't know what she needed.

Nobody else seemed bothered by loud noises or struggled to watch TV. It annoyed her that her friends enjoyed loud restaurants and packed parties while she struggled. She felt like she had nobody to talk to about her communication problems, which weighed on her more and more each day. Once she found other people with hearing loss, the world changed. She saw that she was not alone. She found solace and assistance. She could learn from them. And she did.

Gael grew up with hearing loss. At the time, there were no school programs to assist kids like her, so she did not meet anyone else with similar problems. She lived with hearing loss in a world where everyone else could hear. When she finally met other people like her, she experienced a tremendous release, as if an invisible shell around her cracked open. Like a baby chick, she came into this new world with the sticky residue of past, hidden emotions.

Consider this: *You are not alone in your hearing loss.* It's a monumental health and social issue that is expected to affect one in four people worldwide by 2050, according to the World Health Organization.[7] For every frustration you have with a hearing aid, millions of people have the same issue. And millions more don't have access to even the most basic technology.

Knowing you are not the only one facing these challenges is comforting. They say misery loves company, but it's not the shared misery we seek. Instead, we seek shared *experiences*, the learnings, and the power of the many to impact change.

> **MindShift**
> Many people experience the same challenges as I do. I can learn from them. I'm not alone.

I WANT TO HEAR THE WAY I USED TO

Watching her hearing slip away, audiogram by audiogram—the loss as evident as the ink on the paper—Shari knew that no matter how hard she tried, or how healthily she lived, she could not do anything to reverse the flow. Sometimes this brought her down. It felt hopeless. But then she realized that hearing better does not have to be the goal. She missed the connection to others more than the hearing itself. Once she shifted her focus to communicating better, she was able to apply new skills to enhance her life.

The hard truth is, at this point in time, most types of hearing loss don't have a cure. No medication can repair damaged inner ear hair cells or the auditory nerve. And until that changes, people with sensorineural hearing loss will not be able to hear *exactly* the way they used to. But, when you accept this reality, you may be more willing to use tools that give you the next best thing: effective communication.

MindShift

I want to *communicate* better, and it takes more than hearing aids to do this. I must use other skills and additional technology.

6

HOW TO SHIFT
YOUR MIND

SHARI'S CHILDREN WATCHED their mom trying to hide her hearing loss. They knew she laughed at jokes she had not heard. When Shari realized she was perpetuating the stigma of hearing loss to another generation, she decided it had to stop.

When Gael got her first hearing aid, she tried to hide it, sometimes even using her hand to cover her ear. Now, many years later, she no longer hides her technology. She flaunts it. What she once saw as a big ugly beige piece of plastic and wires, she now sees as two gleaming silvery pieces of magic to be admired.

How do you shift your mind? And how long does it take for transformation to occur?

How well you adapt to change in general is a good indicator of how you do with personal attitude changes. For some, accepting a MindShift and making it part of how they roll takes time and practice. For others, the changes happen like a thunderbolt. But even a flicker of a new outlook can spark confidence that alleviates stress.

Four key strategies can help you change the attitudes that no longer serve you well:

- Optimize rather than perfect

- Practice to build confidence

- Reinforce new attitudes

- Prioritize self-care

OPTIMIZE RATHER THAN PERFECT

Shari is almost as passionate about yoga as she is about hearing loss advocacy. She tries to practice yoga every day, but without access to her regular studio during the pandemic, conditions were not ideal. She created a dedicated space for her yoga practice at home, bringing in space heaters to simulate the warm temperatures of the studio, but her practice was often interrupted by her children walking through to the backyard.

"It's a practice, not a perfect," her yoga teacher reminded the class over Zoom as the students struggled with the frustrations of taking class from home. "Optimize the conditions and do the best you can in the moment. Then try again tomorrow." It's a good mantra for practicing yoga, and it's good advice for living with hearing loss.

In any improvement plan for a listening situation, the most important element is an open-minded attitude. *I'll do my best; but if it doesn't work, we'll try something different next time and, maybe, we'll nail it.*

There are so many communication barriers for people with hearing loss that it doesn't take much to become discouraged. But communication is too fundamental to human happiness to give up on it without a fight. Rather than bemoan poor listening conditions or the ways in which other people are not talking how they're "supposed to," you can focus on what *you* can do to improve the situation. And then do it. In Chapter 16, we detail a simple process called HEAR (hearing check, evaluate, articulate, revise and remind) for assessing and improving every listening situation.

PRACTICE TO BUILD CONFIDENCE

Shari's son was rehearsing for a preschool class recital. He told his mom that his teacher always said that "practice builds confidence."

"Don't you mean practice makes perfect?" Shari asked him.

"No, confidence," he said.

Wise words and an important life lesson that applies to any difficult task. By changing the goal from how well the kids performed to how they felt while rehearsing, the teacher encouraged them to focus on behaviors that led to success.

Developing a better attitude is wonderful, but it only works when you put it into action. For example, if you want to stop hiding and be more open about your hearing loss, you need to practice telling people about it.

It's that simple.

You might hesitate to show off a new attitude, especially with your friends and family. Strangers or people you're meeting for the first time are perfect guinea pigs for your new outlook. Talk to your seatmate on the bus and tell them you have trouble hearing and ask them to speak up, or face you, or whatever you need. Mention it to the cashier who talks to the clothes she's folding rather than to you. Or suggest an alternative communication method to a person mumbling behind a mask.

Practice, practice, practice! It may feel awkward at first, especially if your go-to technique has been to hide, or at least not mention, your hearing loss. But through repetition, self-identifying with hearing loss will soon become your norm—especially when you discover that, most of the time, people are happy to give you what you need.

REINFORCE NEW ATTITUDES

It takes time and patience to break the grip of negative thoughts, and developing a mantra is a good way to crack this barrier. A mantra is simply an affirmation of beliefs. Studies have shown that, when regularly practiced, mantras have positive health benefits.[8]

You give positive reinforcement to *other* people by offering praise, expressing pride in their accomplishments, giving them a high five or a thumbs-up, or even a reward. *Why not do the same for yourself?*

A hearing loss mantra can help you firmly establish a more constructive way of thinking. It can be as easy as regularly saying to yourself, "I've got this!" You can also draw inspiration from the list of MindShifts at the beginning of Chapter 5 (also peppered throughout this book) to create a mantra that works for you. For example: "Hearing loss is just one aspect of who I am. I'm comfortable with myself. I have skills, smarts, and love to share."

Whatever one you choose, try saying it daily, perhaps first thing in the morning. Saying it out loud makes it real. When you can look in the mirror and tell yourself, "There's no shame in having hearing loss, and I am in control," you are seeing the face of positive change.

PRIORITIZE SELF-CARE

Whether we realize it or not—and most of us do—even when we develop a healthier mindset, stress is a by-product of living with hearing loss.

Just to participate in a conversation, especially in a poor listening environment, you must tap into your reserves of mental energy. You may tense up. You may get frustrated. You lipread. You struggle to explain your needs. Stress, stress, stress.

And that stress doesn't disappear after the conversation is finished. It lingers, showing up in many ways. Muscle knots. Poor sleep. Anxiety.

You need to take care of yourself both physically and mentally, and stress reduction is a big part of that. Getting a massage or soaking in a spa are lovely methods of stress relief, but they are not always affordable or available. There are other, less expensive ways to keep stress from boiling over and sabotaging your communication goals.

Keep your energy up! You use an extraordinary amount of energy in your concentration to hear and understand. Without this concentration, you might lose focus and start bluffing. And if you *use* a lot of energy, you need to have it in reserve! Getting enough sleep, eating healthily, and participating in regular exercise provides that energy and improves overall health. In listening situations that require concentration, take occasional breaks to give your eyes (and mind) a rest and to restore your energy.

Gratitude is more than an attitude! Feeling thankful is an active strategy for feeling better. Research shows that feelings of gratitude can benefit our lives through increased patience, better sleep, improved health, higher self-esteem, and more.[9] So, although you might not be grateful for your hearing loss, you *can* be appreciative of the new skill sets that you develop because of it, such as becoming a better communicator. You can offer a thank-you for the amazing hearing technology that transforms your interactions with people you care for. And you can be grateful for all the new sounds you hear or hear *better.* When you take time to *actively* be grateful, the payoff is big.

Find the humor in hearing loss. You probably have at least one funny story about hearing gone wrong. Some hearing "fails" and mis-hears *are* funny, although not always in the moment they happen or to the person with hearing loss. Gael certainly didn't laugh right away when a goofy mutt woke her up to show off his breakfast: her expensive hearing aid, bits of it still hanging out of his mouth. And it didn't seem funny when she accepted a date, only to learn that the man had asked something else entirely. Non sequiturs and mis-hears are always funnier to the *other* person: "Mom, can you help me with an essay?" "That's great, say hi to him for me."

But this was funny right when it happened: At a family dinner, Gael could sense her three-year-old grandson looking up at the side of her head. When she looked down, he smiled and turned his head to reveal the piece of bread crust he'd stuck in *his* ear, an exact replica of Gael's own beige in-the-ear hearing aid. She laughed out loud.

Forgive yourself for less-than-perfect communication. When you tell people about your hearing loss up-front, you give yourself a Get Out of Jail Free card. You don't have to hear perfectly; no one expects it of you, and neither should you. (Similarly, you can cut your communication partners some slack when they are less than perfect.) But there will likely be times when you aren't as open as you should be, when you bluff, when you allow yourself to get frustrated and angry. You will feel relief when you stop holding yourself to an unattainable standard. You owe yourself some self-compassion.

De-stress with proven methods. Earlier, we explored the importance of learning to shift your focus away from the stressors of tinnitus. The same applies to dealing with the emotional strain of hearing loss. Meditation, deep breathing, yoga, and other relaxation techniques offer lasting health benefits. Another important method is writing down your thoughts. Keep a journal to record your feelings about your hearing loss and review them occasionally to see if there have been any changes. And while it sounds clichéd, take up a hobby that doesn't require hearing or communication—painting, perhaps?—anything that allows you to disconnect and decompress.

Respect and protect your residual hearing. Whatever hearing you have, it is precious, valuable—and vulnerable to damage from noise exposure. To protect against further hearing loss, follow these simple guidelines:

- **Move away:** Increasing the distance between you and a loud sound diminishes its impact.

- **Turn it down:** A good rule of thumb is that if you cannot hear someone talking next to you over the music, it is probably too loud.

- **Reduce the time:** Decreasing the duration of your exposure to loud sounds will limit potential damage. Take breaks from the noise to give your ears a rest.

- **Block the sound:** Wear earplugs or earmuffs. Disposable earplugs are available in most drugstores and can be easily carried in a pocket or purse.

To learn more about safe listening levels, ask your HCP.

TECHNOLOGY
Plugging into
Better Hearing

GAEL: Technology can be overwhelming for many people, but I love what it can do for us. Like going from near-deaf to full-on hearing in a nanosecond. When you close the battery cage or press on the sound processor, your world blooms into sound. Gets me almost every time!

 SHARI: How about when you hear a sound—and realize that you've never heard it before? The sound was always there, and others heard it, but to you it didn't exist. Now, with technology, it does.

 GAEL: Hearing aids look so small and simple, but they are powerful and smart enough to be life changing. Talking about this technology makes me teary because it changed *my* life.

 SHARI: Same here. But what excites me even more is all the ways new technologies improve how our hearing aids work! Direct-to-consumer devices and apps, many at a reasonable price or even free, are changing the game of hearing loss tech—all to the benefit of people with hearing loss.

7

BEFRIENDING TECHNOLOGY

WHATEVER YOUR FEELINGS about technology, take a moment to be grateful. Now is the best time ever to have hearing loss. We live in a world of electrically and battery-operated people—a boundary-pushing world where technical dreams are made real every day.

Wearing a small electronic piece is infinitely better than cupping your hand behind your ear or, as was the case a hundred years ago, using an ear trumpet made of shells or animal horns. There was no hiding hearing loss with that!

Why, then, are many people reluctant to adopt ear technology? How have they missed the excitement about today's fantastic hearing electronics?

Many reasons.

Some people feel their hearing loss is not bad enough to warrant the high cost which, for hearing aids, can run into thousands of

You get hearing aids. You take care of them. You put them in and turn them on. And that, my friends, is all I need to know about how hearing aids work.

dollars. Others feel that they're too young—*how could they possibly need a hearing device?* And just about everyone has heard personal anecdotes about technology experiences that didn't go well: too loud, bad fit, squealing, didn't improve hearing.[10]

Denial, anger, or perhaps fear or stigma may fuel the reluctance to adopt technology that occurs on most hearing loss journeys. But the time comes when you realize you must move forward—and hopefully that time came for you, or perhaps that time is now.

> **MindShift**
> Technology is my friend. My devices let me hear sounds I had forgotten or had never heard before. They connect me to other people and the world.

The technology boom in assistive devices is exciting. Regardless of how mild or profound your loss, you have options that include a new wave of hearing aid designs and accessories, cochlear implants, and direct-to-consumer options like hearables and apps. Change is occurring so rapidly that between the time of writing and the moment you read these words, a crop of new options will most likely have been introduced.

If you have not yet tried assistive technology, or if you tried hearing aids but then threw them in a drawer, we encourage you to give hearing technology a role in your life.

FOUR CATEGORIES OF HEARING TECHNOLOGY

You may already be in love with how hearing technology can change your life. And like us, you may also be overwhelmed at times by the sheer volume of choice. Choosing the right device—or mix of devices—for your way of living requires some research, as do most life-enhancing purchases. You may also need the support of a communication specialist such as an HCP who understands the full range of hearing technology. Your hearing loss peers and online forums are also great sources of new technology ideas.

The first three categories of hearing technology comprise *personal technologies* that you wear or use to connect yourself with the world of sound, while the fourth relates to *external accommodations*: larger-scale technologies that create a hearing-accessible environment for everyone.

We group personal technologies based on how you access the product:

- **Hearing clinics:** You order devices through a hearing care provider.

- **Direct-to-consumer (DTC):** You purchase products directly from a store or website.

- **Smartphone apps:** You download the technology directly onto your phone.

Devices and programs in these groups have some overlap. For example, you can buy hearing aids from either an HCP or an online outlet.

You may use products from all three personal technology categories. For example, your HCP-acquired hearing aids may connect to a hearing app on your smartphone or a TV device purchased online. Or you may use a speech-to-text app on your phone to fill in the words your hearing aids don't pick up in a difficult listening environment.

The fourth category of hearing technology, external accommodations, includes large-scale technologies like hearing loops and CART (*Communication Access Realtime Translation*, where a trained captioner transcribes spoken words into readable text), which are used in public spaces, the workplace, educational and medical situations, and anywhere you need assistance to hear and communicate better.

If you've never heard about hearing loops or CART, you are not alone. Your authors didn't know about either of these miraculous technologies for many years for a simple reason: our HCPS never mentioned them. It wasn't until each of us attended our first hearing loss convention that we experienced the technologies in action and realized that, in many ways, society could be providing better access for people with hearing loss.

In the coming chapters, we do a deep dive on each of these four categories of technology.

8

DEVICES FROM HEARING CARE PROFESSIONALS

A N HCP IS the first stop for most people with hearing loss. An audiologist or a hearing instrument specialist will help you choose appropriate hearing technology, with a focus on three main types:

- hearing aids
- cochlear implants (CIs)
- accessories (often brand specific)

HEARING AIDS: THE PRIMARY WORKHORSE (FOR MOST)

The process of obtaining hearing aids has not changed much in decades. Depending on the rules and regulations in your area, you may be referred to an HCP by a family doctor or an ENT, or you may book a hearing evaluation directly with an HCP.

HCPs undergo years of training in hearing and hearing loss and should recommend a hearing aid with the technical and style features that are best for you. One caution: Work with an HCP that sells a variety of styles and brands so you are not limited in your choices. If they sell only one brand of hearing aid, find another HCP.

Once your hearing aids arrive from the manufacturer, your HCP will program them to your individual needs, based on your audiogram and lifestyle preferences. For example, if you have dexterity issues, a rechargeable battery will be important. Devices may also be set up with alternate programs that change the hearing aid settings for different listening situations. For example, a restaurant program may be helpful in loud, reverberant spaces, or a music program might enhance the sound of music.

New supplemental programs for hearing aids are continually being developed. For example, during the pandemic, hearing aid manufacturers and HCPs created face mask programs to boost the higher-pitched speech sounds that masks block, making it easier to understand speech, even from behind a face mask.

CHOOSING THE RIGHT HEARING AIDS

If you thought deciding to get a hearing aid was the hardest part of the whole process, it probably was! But now you need to focus on which one to get.

Putting a price on hearing is impossible, but the purchase of hearing aids often forces us to do exactly that because they tend to be expensive. Should someone have to save up for a hearing aid, a necessary health device, with proven psycho-social benefits? We save up for a new condo or a new car. We should not have to save up for something as crucial to our health as a hearing aid! But since insurance schemes in many countries do not cover hearing aids, we are forced to do so or go without. For this reason, direct-to-consumer and other lower-cost options are increasingly attractive to people with certain types of hearing loss.

Before deciding where to spend your resources, you need to understand what hearing aids can and cannot do. Hearing aids are modern miracle devices, but they are not a silver bullet. People often expect hearing aids to "cure" their hearing problems, to correct hearing loss in the way that wearing glasses corrects vision. With these expectations, many people get a rude shock.

Success with hearing aid technology depends on many factors, including the degree and type of hearing loss, the presence of other hearing-related issues such as tinnitus, and the use of additional technical and non-technical communication strategies. Just as influential are personality, lifestyle, and—we know you're expecting this—attitude!

Hearing aids cannot replicate the body's natural, perfect hearing ability. Because of this, they *cannot*:

- deliver sounds as sharply as heard by the natural ear

- read your mind—they amplify all sounds rather than just those you want to hear

- distinguish among numerous simultaneous speakers

- block out all unwanted background noise

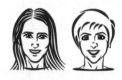

Two must-have features in hearing aids are telecoils and streaming capability via Bluetooth.

Hearing aids *can*:

- improve speech comprehension, especially in a quiet environment

- reduce (but not eliminate) listening effort and fatigue

- improve personal speech clarity and volume (because you hear yourself better)

- assist with sound localization

- mask or reduce the effects of tinnitus

- connect to other devices to enhance communication

- combine with non-technical strategies, such as lipreading, to improve speech comprehension

Hearing aids vary in size, shape, color, and how they fit in the ear. Decades of research and technological developments have gone into creating sleek and sophisticated devices that provide an increasingly improved sound experience. This ongoing and innovative research is part of what makes the devices so expensive.

Do Your Research

Choosing a hearing aid is like any serious, major purchase—what's right for me might not be right for you. Although you will discuss the decision with an expert—your HCP—doing some outside research is a good idea as well.

Visit hearing aid review websites that show the full feature comparisons of different models and their accessories, and see what users are saying about the pros and cons of different devices. Reach out to your hearing loss peers or visit social media groups to learn what features are most critical to other users. (Ignore the Negative Nelly types and focus on relevant feedback.)

Then think about your lifestyle and the situations where enhanced hearing is most important to you. The intersection of these two is your sweet spot. Discuss your findings with your hearing professional—and together you can pick a winner!

We are often asked which brand is the best or if we recommend a particular hearing aid. Over the years, we've used many, because our hearing has changed and hearing aids just keep getting better and better. More important than any specific brand is having a skilled HCP who insists on your input at all stages of the process of fitting a hearing aid.

Style Options

Every few years, Shari takes a new pair of hearing aids out for a spin to see if the updated features are worth the extra cost. Sometimes she upgrades, other times she sticks with what is already working for her. She likes to know what's out there, and she doesn't want to miss out on something spectacular.

The degree and type of your hearing loss will influence the decision on hearing aid style. Devices are designed to look good—consider what an "attractive hearing aid" might mean for you—and to address the requirements of your hearing loss. The smallest hearing aids may not be adequate for severe losses.

The most popular style today is an open-fit, behind-the-ear hearing aid, with a barely visible tube going into the ear. Various styles of in-the-canal aids are less visible but, again, not all styles deliver the necessary amplification and functionality for certain hearing losses. View the options online to get a feel for your choices, which you can then discuss with your service provider.

Shari has always worn hearing aids that are designed to sit deep in her ear canal. At first this was because of the stigma she felt about getting hearing aids, but she stuck with them out of habit and because she likes how they help her locate where sounds originate.

Gael has worn just about every style going, starting with a series of behind-the-ear models, then in-the-canal, in-the-ear, and now back to behind-the-ear. When she started wearing two aids, she called the left one Billy and the right one Bob. But now that she's bimodal—using a hearing aid in one ear and a cochlear implant on the other side—she needs new names. Perhaps Thing 1 and Thing 2?

Bells and Whistles

Gael's hearing loss was mild as a child, becoming severe to profound in her thirties. As her hearing worsened, she could actually hear better and better thanks to continually improving hearing aid technology.

Hearing aids have amazing, high-tech sounding features which may be useful to you, depending on your type and degree of hearing loss and lifestyle. These features include rechargeable batteries, directional microphones, tinnitus masking, extra noise reduction, remote controls, wireless streaming, and *telecoils* (commonly known as *T-coils*)—small wires in a hearing device that let you connect to a hearing loop. Features such as embedded fitness trackers or fall detection may add more to the cost than to the functionality. Discuss these options with your HCP.

Two must-have features in hearing aids are T-coils and streaming capability via Bluetooth, both of which bring sound directly into your devices. To accommodate both, the hearing aid may need to be slightly larger, but the universal connectivity they provide is worth the increase in size.

The T-coil in a hearing aid or sound processor connects the device to induction hearing loops and hearing aid–compatible telephones. Bluetooth connectivity allows wireless streaming to almost any electronic device. When you connect your aids to other devices via Bluetooth, you can watch TV, stream videos, participate in video conference calls, and take phone calls—all with the sound coming directly into your aids.

Your HCP may promote Bluetooth over T-coils (and may neglect to mention telecoils at all), but you need *both* technologies since they are used in different situations. Bluetooth works for streaming via personal devices like laptops, smartphones, and TV sets, or for public devices such as the audio-guides used in museums and art galleries. But hearing loop systems for T-coils are more commonly found in public places like theaters or at conferences and lecture halls, and T-coils are in most public telephones—if you can find one!

It is important to ask your HCP to activate the T-coil and explain how to use it in a variety of settings. If your current hearing aid doesn't have one, you may be able to get a telecoil-equipped accessory that works with your hearing aid. Ask your provider to include a T-coil in your new or next round of hearing aids.

Test Driving

You wouldn't buy a new car without taking it for a test drive, and you wouldn't buy new clothes without trying them on. The same goes for hearing aids; you may need to try different styles or brands to see which one sounds and feels the best to you. Providers must offer a trial period of *at least* thirty days, during which you can test the hearing aids in your usual listening situations, including group conversations, which are often the most challenging. If you are not offered a trial period, find another provider.

After the initial fitting, your HCP may need to adjust the programming or the fit of the earpiece. If you decide you want to forgo hearing aids for a while, you can return them, usually with a small restocking fee. If your hearing loss is mild to moderate, a direct-to-consumer device may suffice.

Training Your Brain

When you start wearing a hearing aid, your brain needs time to adjust to the new sound information it is receiving. Things may seem *loud* for a while. The high frequency *s* and *sh* may seem extremely hissy. But soon your brain will interpret this as normal, and you will be aware of hearing better. That is why, during the trial period, it's important to wear your hearing aids as much as possible and in many different situations.

Here's the catch. If you decide you want to try a different hearing aid, you will go through a similar adjustment period—because the brain must once again adjust to new information. The sound input varies between brands, technologies, and styles. By the time your brain has adapted to the second hearing aid, it may be difficult to remember how things sounded with the first one! You can't play back and easily compare the brain's interpretations. You may try the second one and say *yes!* Or you may think the first one was better, or maybe you need something completely different. Your HCP is trained to help you through this challenging process to make the best possible choice. Your job is to keep an open mind and to ask all the questions you need.

I BOUGHT MY HEARING AIDS: NOW WHAT?

The day she got her first hearing aid was a big one for Gael and her family. At twenty, she had been waiting a long time for something that her doctors said wouldn't help. But finally, a new physician had a different opinion and prescribed a hearing aid.

The hearing aid dispenser's clinic was on a busy, booming street. As she left the clinic, being told to "go forth and hear" (seriously), Gael was assaulted with noise. As she walked the few city blocks to her father's office, she lurched and spun along the sidewalk, recoiling at car horns and the screeching brakes of the streetcars. When she reached his office, her father's welcoming smile disappeared as Gael broke down in tears. After twenty years of relative quiet, the intense loudness was a shock to Gael's system. But after a couple of false starts, she fell in love with her hearing aid and all the others that followed.

Getting new hearing aids is exciting, although we admit it includes an element of "no pain, no gain." It's not like getting a new car, where you pay for it, fill the tank, buckle up, and then step on the gas and away you go. Breaking in hearing aids is more like taking dance lessons with a new partner. You and your hearing aids have to get used to each other. There will be a lot of smashing into each other, painful foot-crunches, and wanting to go in opposite directions. It takes more than a few lessons before the bumbling becomes a smooth tango. Your HCP is like a dance instructor, performing a series of tweaks on the fit, the venting, the volume, the programs, the highs, the lows, and whatever is needed to make the dance enjoyable and successful.

How quickly and well you adapt to your first or twentieth set of hearing aids depends on:

- how much you want them

- the severity of your hearing loss

- how well you understand the various settings, when used alone and when connecting to other devices

- how much patience you have when you don't understand how to use them

- your manual dexterity in performing tasks such as changing small batteries and even tinier wax guards

- having realistic expectations—hearing aids are powerful devices, but they will not meet all your communication needs

GET THE MOST OUT OF YOUR HEARING AIDS

"I can hear better than when I could hear!" A friend was trying to describe to Gael what his new hearing aids had given back to him. He had put off getting them for years, and his newfound level of hearing seemed better than at any point in his life.

Hearing aids may be miraculous life-changing devices, but they still require love, tenderness, and methodical care to perform optimally. Here are some tips for getting the most out of them.

Wear Them Every Day!

Your hearing aids can't help you hear if they have been stuffed in a drawer. Wear your hearing aids all day, every day for maximum benefit and to keep your brain stimulated. Your HCP may suggest a gradual breaking-in process, but the sooner you get to full-time use, the sooner your brain will adapt. Although taking them off in the quiet of your home is tempting, remember that a home is rarely completely quiet. You may need to relearn the sounds of many little house noises—the hum of a fridge, the whirr of air vents, or the cat scratching at the door. Take your aids out only for showering and sleeping.

You will likely be intensely aware of your hearing aids at first, but wearing them shouldn't be painful. When fitted properly, they should feel weightless and motionless in the ear, with almost no intrusion into your thoughts or actions. If you do experience pain or discomfort, they need an adjustment by your HCP. Over time, they will become so comfortable you may even forget you're wearing them.

Sometimes the extreme comfort of hearing aids can get you into trouble. Because you don't feel them, you're not aware of them. Gael was in the shower and with the thought, "I've never heard the water so clearly before," she almost smashed through the shower door in her panic to get out!

Involve Your Family

Communication is a two-way activity. Your hearing loss affects your family and friends, too. As you go through the process of getting used to hearing aids, it helps to recognize *their* unique frustrations. It's not easy living with a loved one who's undergoing a brain transformation (which *is* what you're going through).

Unless your partner or other family members are also hearing aid users, they won't understand the process of breaking in a hearing aid, especially for the first time. Expressing how *loud* everything is and explaining your frustrations in a way that doesn't make them feel guilty or equally frustrated can be challenging. When your family better understands hearing loss, and specifically *your* hearing loss, they will be better at empathizing with you and supporting you.

Learn About Your Hearing Aid Features

You want to get maximum benefit from your valuable equipment. Take the time to understand the various settings on your hearing aids and what they can do for you. What's the point of having exciting listening features if you don't use them?

Hearing aid manuals tend to be generic, but "how-to" videos are easy to find online, including those on manufacturers' websites. They can be lifesaving.

Take Care of Them

Regular home maintenance includes removing gunk out of air vents and changing the wax guards, because sound is crisper when it's not fighting its way through *cerumen*, the pretty name for earwax. Wipe down the aid's surface from time to time and change the open-fit tips when necessary. Do *not* try to repair your own hearing aids—it won't end well. Schedule regular visits—every six months or so—at the hearing clinic for internal cleaning and maintenance.

Your hearing devices can withstand a lot of abuse (you should see how they test them at the manufacturing stage), but any trauma should be accidental. Dropping them or almost drowning them in the shower is forgivable, and usually the devices bounce back with a bit of coaxing. But grinding them beneath your heel is just an expensive temper tantrum.

Almost everyone has a hearing aid horror story, and Gael has several. But which one to tell first? You've heard about the dog that ate her hearing aid. And when she almost drowned her aid in the shower. But what about when she grabbed the pull string of her in-the-canal aid to show it to a group of audiology students and only the top half came out? The bottom half stayed in her ear, and they all stared in horror at the wires hanging from Gael's precious hearing aid as tears sprung to her eyes. She thought it would be a funny story someday, but it still isn't.

Keep Them Dry

Moisture is enemy number one to your sensitive devices. One of the most important things you can do is to put your hearing aids in a drying aid *every night*. Drying aids come in many sizes, including small ones designed for traveling, and should be available from your HCP. After showering or swimming, give your ears a half hour to dry before putting your aids back in. If your aid gets an unexpected soaking, dry it off, open the battery cage, and place it in the drying aid for a few hours. If you don't have access to a proper drying aid, try placing it in a plastic container with uncooked rice. If it still doesn't work, don't panic; pull yourself together and call your HCP.

Stay in Touch with Your HCP

Your hearing aids need regular professional TLC. So do you. Schedule annual visits to test your hearing, ask questions, and see if any programming changes are available or needed. At the same time, your HCP will clean up your devices, check for wear and tear, and ensure all parts are working the way they should.

Don't ignore your hearing health—it's an important part of your overall good health. At any time, if you feel something has changed with your hearing, or your devices don't seem to be at the top of their game, contact your HCP. They will want to hear from you when this happens. It bears repeating that *if your hearing level drops suddenly, this is a medical emergency.* Call your doctor or head to the emergency room right away.

COCHLEAR IMPLANTS: THE MIRACLE OF HEARING RESTORATION

Sometimes hearing aids are just not strong enough to provide the necessary amplification.

As Gael's hearing worsened, there was always better hearing aid technology to help her. She knew many people whose lives had changed dramatically with cochlear implants, but she had been told she wouldn't qualify because she functioned so highly with hearing aids. Secretly, she was pleased. Then a new audiologist looked at her audiogram and said, "Why don't you have a cochlear implant?" Like many people, she had been telling herself that she was doing just fine with her hearing aids, but in reality it was time for the next step.

Usable hearing, also called *residual hearing,* can decrease to the point that amplification through even the most powerful hearing aids does not provide sufficient understanding of speech or environmental sounds. This used to be the end of the road, metaphorically speaking, for people with this degree of deafness. There was nothing more that could be done.

Then, in the 1980s, a scientific breakthrough! Hearing scientists discovered that the road did keep going—with the cochlear implant (CI), a modern miracle of hearing.

The human cochlea has fifteen thousand hair cells, give or take a few, that are crucial to the hearing process. When too many hair cells become damaged—for any of a number of reasons, including disease, genetics, acoustic trauma, or noise exposure—permanent hearing loss occurs.

The cochlear implant procedure replaces the damaged hair cells with an electrical array inserted into the cochlea. When the implant is activated, an external processor collects sound and transmits it directly to an internal receiver, which sends electrical impulses along the auditory nerve to the brain. Just as in natural hearing, the brain translates this information into recognizable sounds—someone laughing or rain plopping in the puddles.

When Gael returned home the day her CI was activated, she asked her husband, also known as the Hearing Husband, "What's that sound?" He asked her to describe it.

"*Nyok-nyok-nyok.*"

"It's the clock!" he said. "Hey, everybody, Gael can hear the clock!"

"That's nice," she said. "Now, could you turn it down?"

After implantation, it takes time for the brain to adapt to this different type of information. As a crucial part of a successful acclimation process, CI recipients learn how to listen to and understand these new sounds with daily practice and exercises. Gradually, as CI users improve their listening skills, environmental noises, initially perceived as screeches and whistles, start to make sense and sound "normal." All speech, regardless of who is talking, sounds like Donald Duck at first, but with practice, the CI user learns to differentiate between a spouse, a parent, and a child.

In many countries, CIs are now fully covered by insurance, but access to cochlear implants is not universal. It is a costly medical procedure, and receiving one is limited by a government's willingness to provide it or health insurance to cover it. As more health jurisdictions accept cochlear implants as a medical necessity for people with severe to profound hearing loss, we hope to see them become more widely available.

If you are interested in a cochlear implant, your HCP can evaluate whether you are a candidate and, if you are, refer you for further assessments.

ACCESSORIES: PERFORMANCE ENHANCERS FOR YOUR DEVICES

Hearing aids don't always perform well in noisy settings or when you are far away from the speaker. Hearing aid accessories to the rescue!

These performance enhancers are useful in any situation where you want to bring sound directly into your ears, especially in noisy situations such as professional meetings, at the dinner table, traveling in the car, watching TV, or streaming movies on the computer. There are a broad range of accessories, including remote microphones, streamers, and neck loops that use either Bluetooth or telecoil connection depending on the situation.

Most hearing aid manufacturers offer these accessories for an extra fee, but unfortunately, they are brand specific. Down the road, if you change brands, you may need to replace your accessories, too.

Advocates have urged manufacturers to adopt a common standard for accessories so they work interchangeably across brands. Because of the expense, some consumers, especially those with mild to moderate hearing loss, are opting to use more universal solutions like apps instead.

9

DIRECT-TO-CONSUMER DEVICES

AFTER DECADES OF a single delivery model for hearing devices through the HCP channel, change is happening. Hearing technologies of various styles and price points are now (or may soon be) available—direct to you, the consumer with hearing loss. While direct-to-consumer (DTC) devices are often geared towards people with mild to moderate hearing loss—the assumption being that this group can do without the expertise and involvement of an HCP—the proliferation of choices will benefit all of us, no matter what degree of loss we have. Competition creates innovation and lowers prices. Both have already begun.

DTC devices fall into four general categories:

- hearing aids
- hearables
- amplifiers
- alerting devices

DIRECT-TO-CONSUMER HEARING AIDS

Currently DTC hearing aids are available for purchase online, but the quality is mixed. They are in a gray category for regulation, so while some are safe and effective to use, others are not. Read customer and professional reviews carefully, and if something seems too good to be true or too cheap to be good, it probably is. However, some quality DTC hearing aids offer remote programming by an HCP as well as follow-up care appointments. Some may also include linked accessories. Depending on the complexity and severity of your hearing loss, DTC hearing aids can be workable options, and price points are highly competitive. Reputable outfits will allow a minimum thirty-day trial period before the sale is final.

A soon-to-be-available sub-category of DTC hearing aids in the United States, termed *over-the-counter hearing aids*, would be sold through pharmacies, other brick-and-mortar stores, and online. Appropriate for people with perceived mild to moderate hearing loss, these self-fitting devices, unlike current DTC hearing aids, would be regulated for safety and efficacy by a government agency. Depending on consumer uptake, these products could also become available worldwide. Lower prices may also trickle slowly into the traditional channel, benefitting us all.

HEARABLES: "FRIENDS WITH BENEFITS"

Hearables are devices, usually earbuds or headphones, that offer *hearing enhancement* through amplification, noise cancellation, and other smart technology that increases hearing ability. Often their primary function is streaming music or movies, and they are usually targeted at people with typical hearing, not hearing loss.

But because of the amplification and noise-cancellation capabilities, hearables—particularly those that incorporate sound personalization via an online or device-based hearing test—can also be useful for people with certain types of hearing loss.

Hearables are most often purchased through retail outlets or online, but some forward-thinking HCPs carry them as well. Although some hearables can be worn all day like a traditional hearing aid, most have limited battery life—less than a full day of continuous use—and are designed to be worn only in certain listening situations. Some, like Apple AirPods Pro, use the iPhone's built-in microphone to pick up the sound, while others may require linking to a smartphone app. Hearables can also be good back-up devices for people with mild to moderate hearing loss, and possibly for those with even more severe losses.

The rise of hearables has additional benefits. The more "normal" it becomes for people to take advantage of hearing assistance, in whatever form and even if only in certain situations, the more the stigma surrounding hearing loss and hearing technology will wither away.

AMPLIFIERS: SIMPLE SOLUTIONS IN A PINCH

Personal sound amplification products (PSAPs) are wearable listening products intended to amplify sounds for people who do not have hearing loss. They are usually marketed for use in certain situations—for example, while hunting or birding—where superhuman hearing is helpful. They are not intended for all-day use.

Although not usually designed for people with hearing loss, PSAPs can be used to amplify speech if no better option exists. For example, some PSAPs are effective in hospitals and other medical settings for communicating with patients with hearing loss who do not have their own devices. A PSAP can also be used as a back-up device in a pinch should your primary hearing device be on the fritz.

ALERTING DEVICES: BE SAFE AND INDEPENDENT

How does a person with hearing loss, traveling alone, get up on time when staying in a hotel? It's not easy. Because you don't hear the phone, wake-up calls are useless. A portable alerting device that either turns on the lights or vibrates to shake you awake might work. If Gael needs to get up for an early flight, she often wakes up frequently during the night, worrying that her alerting device will fail her. It hasn't happened yet, but the best solution for her is to not book an early flight!

People with hearing loss don't *do* auditory alerts. Sure, you *might* hear the fire alarm—but who wants to take that risk? To hear doorbells, phones, and crying babies, you need something more: a super-loud tone, or visual or tactile alerts.

Making It Louder

If you can't hear an alert, one option is to make it louder. Telephones, doorbells, and alarm clocks often come with adjustable volume. Amplified alerts can be very loud—up to one hundred decibels or more when activated. Several brands of landline telephones offer this type of product. Extra-loud ringtones are also available for most smartphones.

But loud tone alerts can be disruptive to others and possibly dangerous. They can damage residual hearing, particularly for people close to the alert speaker. According to the National Institute on Deafness and other Communication Disorders, two minutes of exposure to sounds at 110 dB or more can cause permanent hearing loss.[11]

Visual Alerts

A better option may be a visual alert, where a sound at normal volume triggers a secondary alert of a flashing or strobe light. This method works well for doorbells, telephone ringers, and baby monitors, as well as already loud alerts like fire alarms and other emergency notifications. Some auditory alert systems have a visual alert option built in and both are activated simultaneously. Others are separate units you place next to the speaker of the audible alert. When a tone is detected, a separate visual signal is activated. Depending on the size of your home, you may need multiple receivers so that you can see the flash in every room.

Tactile Alerts

Vibration alerts work well for alarm clocks, baby monitors, and for any situation when an auditory or visual alert doesn't work. Place a vibrating pad under your mattress or pillow to be shaken awake. You can also set up tactile alerts from your smartphone to a smartwatch or exercise tracker. When you link them, a phone call or text message will jiggle your wrist.

Both Apple and Android phones include sound recognition alerts built into the operating systems. Enable the feature in your phone's accessibility settings and your phone will vibrate whenever it detects one of the sounds you select for monitoring. Choices include a variety of alarms (fire, siren, smoke), household sounds (doorbells, door knocking, water running) as well as animal sounds and human sounds like a baby crying.

WHY CARE ABOUT DTC OPTIONS?

If you have severe hearing loss, DTC devices likely won't serve your needs. You will probably require more sophisticated devices, skilled professionals to finetune your settings, multiple programs, and linked hearing assistive technologies that may not yet be available in DTC offerings.

Still, DTC products are exciting for many reasons:

- People with mild to moderate hearing loss, who may not otherwise treat their hearing loss, may adopt DTC devices earlier.

- DTC devices make good back-ups for emergencies.

- Technological advances from DTC devices may be incorporated into more traditional hearing aids and vice versa.

- Increased competition may drive down prices for traditional devices.

- As more people wear cool-looking things in their ears, awareness of hearing loss will grow and the stigma often associated with the use of hearing assistance will fade.

Even more exciting, with competition from other sales channels, we see the role of the hearing care professional evolving into that of a communication specialist who provides a broad scope of hearing services to meet the needs of clients.

BUYER, BEWARE

The case for making lower cost, mass-produced technology available is compelling. The cost of traditional hearing aids, which must be replaced every few years, is staggering, often with little to no financial support from government or private health systems. Many potential users don't "see the value" in hearing aids, meaning they don't see the potential benefits as worth the high cost.

But there are risks to eliminating trained hearing professionals from the process. Without professional guidance, there is a higher risk that the devices could be used improperly, providing too much or too little amplification. Also, while some DTC devices are safe and effective, others are not, and it may be hard for the consumer to tell the difference.

We strongly encourage meeting with a hearing care professional as one of the first steps when you suspect hearing loss. Even if you don't buy technology from them, a proper diagnosis will help you make a better technology decision.

If DTC options appeal to you, check online reviews, do research via user forums, and use common sense. Be aware that trial periods and return policies may differ. Ask your HCP for recommendations; the best service providers will be familiar with at least some of the options.

10

USING APPS TO HELP YOU HEAR

OW DID WE live before we had apps?

Apps, the short form of *applications,* are software programs that run on devices to keep you organized, fit, entertained... and to hear? Hearing scientists and the tech geniuses have collaborated, sometimes with spectacular results, to harness hearing devices to smart technology, making lives infinitely easier.

The most basic type of app comes with your hearing aids, linking them to your smartphone. Your HCP does the initial setup, but from then on you control a variety of hearing aid settings. Typically, you can adjust the volume and switch between programs such as a T-coil or a music program or connect to accessories like a TV streamer, a remote mic, and personal devices. You can check battery status and set up alerts for when a hearing aid battery is about to die. You can adjust the level of treble and bass, apply noise filters, and even locate your misplaced hearing aid under a pile of clothes!

But even more exciting are two categories of apps designed to improve your hearing and communication: *speech-to-text apps* and *amplifier apps*.

SPEECH-TO-TEXT APPS

Some people love captions and look for them everywhere—even where they aren't. Gael knows a woman who, in an argument with her husband, looked at the TV to see if, by some miracle, his words were showing up on the screen! At her daughter's high school plays, Shari's eyes involuntarily glided to the side of the stage looking for the caption screen anytime she missed some of the dialogue. The play was not captioned, but her "caption reflex" made her laugh.

Of all the apps available to people with hearing loss, the most exciting are speech-to-text apps, which translate the spoken word into something you can read. This type of captioning uses automatic speech recognition (ASR), and the quality and speed are improving every day. The text is similar to the captions that appear at the bottom of television screens, but they are created in real-time through computer processing.

Many of these apps were originally designed for creating transcripts and note-taking during business meetings. But the hearing loss population has embraced them with joy! It doesn't take long to find the necessary and natural balance between watching a person's face and reading their words on the phone.

Speech-to-text apps are useful at almost any time—in meetings, on video conference calls, at lectures, and even in noisy situations. Any place where your phone's microphone can detect the spoken word, it can translate it into a written form.

My hearing aids died on an overseas trip, and I learned the importance of having a back-up plan. Alternative hearing technologies saved the day.

Captioning apps are not yet perfect, but the quality is improving rapidly. An external microphone attached to your smartphone can help it better "hear" the dialogue for easier translation and increased accuracy.

AMPLIFIER APPS TO THE RESCUE

Amplifier apps work like personal sound amplification products (PSAPs) but use your smartphone as a directional microphone. Access the sound by pairing your smartphone and hearing aids or by using earbuds or headphones. This type of app is a good tool for medical appointments, lectures, meetings, or in restaurants— anytime or anywhere you need a volume boost. Amplifier apps are especially helpful for people with milder losses who may not (yet) be using hearing aids, but they can also be useful for hearing aid users in noisy environments or as a back-up communication tool when hearing devices become unexpectedly damaged or broken.

On an overseas trip, both of Shari's hearing aids died, leaving her the *deafest* she had ever been. Yet there were still ten more days of touring planned. New devices or a quick repair were not an option seven thousand miles from home.

She reached out to her hearing loss network for suggestions and quickly learned about several apps that would let her use her iPhone microphone as a hearing aid. She purchased a pair of in-ear noise-cancelling headphones and used them in combination with an amplifier app.

Although it was not perfect, this workaround allowed her to hear the tour guides (as long as she was standing close to them and pointing her phone's microphone at them) and converse with her traveling companions at meals. Using an amplifier app saved the trip.

11

EXTERNAL ACCOMMODATIONS

H OW CAN SOCIETY help you hear?
No new building, airport, or other public space is constructed without including ramps for people who use wheelchairs. But these ramps are also beneficial for people with other mobility challenges and people pushing baby strollers or carrying heavy luggage.

Accessible design works for everyone—including people living with hearing loss. When public places and entertainment venues include hearing loops or other listening systems and visual assistance such as captioning and signage, we can understand speeches, theater performances, courtroom dialogue, and announcements at the airport. Accessible design works for hearing people who also struggle with garbled airport PA announcements.

Today, accessibility for people with hearing loss in public spaces is still limited, but with advocacy efforts and the enforcement of local accessibility laws, it is slowly changing for the better.

The more we ask for accommodations at large events, museums, and other venues, the more familiar the general public will be with the options that exist and the more likely that other venues will offer them as well. Half the battle is that many people with hearing loss don't know about these options. The other half is getting up our individual nerve to ask for what we need. You're reading this— so now you know what's out there. From now on, you can ask for it!

> **MindShift**
> It is my right to ask for and receive equal access. When I advocate for myself, I am also creating change that benefits others.

The most common and effective accommodations for use in public spaces are:

- captioning
- hearing loops
- alternative listening systems
- caption readers for theaters

CAPTIONING

Captioning benefits are not limited to people with hearing loss. They are powerful development and learning tools for people with auditory processing disorders and for second-language learners. Captions make it easier to understand complicated or confusing content and improve intelligibility of a fast talker or speaker with a strong accent. Captioned content also engages viewers for longer periods and is easier to remember.[12]

There are two basic delivery methods. The first is Communication Access Realtime Translation, or CART, which is like closed captioning on TV, but is provided in real time, with a person transcribing speech as it is uttered, on screens set up for this purpose. CART is a phonetically produced technology that originated in the courtroom, with stenographers recording every spoken word of proceedings—accurately and quickly. The process has been adapted for people with hearing loss.

When used for hearing accommodation, CART captioners are required to caption *all* speech, unlike lower-cost forms of text interpretation, such as computer note taking, that summarize a person's words. People with hearing loss have the right to receive the full message as uttered by the speaker. Some conference setups even offer CART on personal devices.

At Gael's first group meeting with other people who had hearing loss, she was the guest speaker. As she stood at the podium talking, her eyes kept flitting to the miracle on the screen beside her, where, via CART, her words appeared just a second after she spoke them! After asking the audience for a moment to herself, she turned and talked to the screen, and it perfectly displayed her words back at her. Everyone laughed, but for Gael, it was the first of many life-changing moments to come.

CART is a wonderful accommodation, but it can be expensive—up to $200 or more per hour, depending on the location and quality of the captioner. In many countries, CART is a qualified accommodation that can be requested in a work or educational setting. CART can also be requested at public meetings and at theater and other performances.

The second type of captioning is automatic speech recognition, or ASR captions. Earlier we described how ASR captioning fuels personal speech-to-text apps. This same technology can be used to caption video conference calls and webinars and any video content posted on a website or social media platform, including YouTube.

When the pandemic hit, many holiday celebrations moved online. Spotty internet connections and poor computer microphones made it hard for Shari to participate. Luckily, her family was willing to experiment with a variety of video conferencing platforms to find one that had high-quality ASR captions. The transcription wasn't perfect, but it helped her fill in some of the dialogue she was missing.

Once you become accustomed to ASR captions, you'll likely note the mistakes—such as when the word *merely* is transcribed as *merrily*—and mentally correct them to fit the context of the conversation. Jargon and specialized terms can be a problem, however, since the artificial intelligence may not have encountered them before. This is a current advantage of CART, where specific terms and names can be preprogrammed for a captioning event. Hopefully, ASR captions will soon offer this capability as well.

ASR captions are becoming more widespread. At this writing, Google has added automatic captioning to all video content viewed in its Chrome browser when its Live Caption feature is enabled in the Accessibility settings. Other browsers and social media platforms are likely to follow.

Because ASR captioning is not yet 100 percent accurate, it may not be the best choice when accuracy is mandated, such as in legal situations and many educational, medical, or work settings. But for personal communications or a meeting of a local club or panel discussion hosted by a small nonprofit with no budget for CART, ASR captions are rapidly becoming an effective and inexpensive alternative.

HEARING LOOPS

Another life-changing moment: The first time Gael put her hearing aids on T-coil mode at a hearing loss conference, she was shocked to tears. The speaker was a hundred feet away on the stage, but his voice flowed directly into Gael's hearing aids.

Another time, she entered from the back of the huge ballroom, and as she stepped over the wire of the hearing loop, Gael could hear the speaker as clearly as if she were standing beside her. She stepped back over the wire ... no sound. Stepped in ... sound. Out again ... silence. Someone saw her doing what must have looked like a very slow dance with herself and asked her if she was alright. "Yes," Gael answered. "Just enjoying a miracle."

A hearing loop, also called an audio induction loop, uses electromagnetism to create a wireless audio signal that is picked up by hearing devices in the T-coil setting when they are within the circle of a wire loop. When properly set up and maintained, the system closes the gap between speaker and listener, eliminating most background noise and restoring the intimacy of sound, speech, and music that for many was lost along with their hearing.

Large-room hearing loops work well for lectures and speeches, as well as theater and music performances. Smaller loop systems are used in banks and at hotel check-in counters, and even for your own TV! Personal neck loops can transmit sound from devices such as a cellphone into hearing aids and cochlear implant sound processors.

ALTERNATIVE LISTENING SYSTEMS

Although not as convenient as hearing loops, FM and infrared systems are the traditional accessibility options used in public spaces and entertainment venues.

FM systems use radio signals to transmit sounds. Speakers wear a microphone connected to a transmitter that sends the sound to an FM-linked device tuned to a specific frequency. FM systems can transmit signals up to three hundred feet, so they work well in public spaces.

Infrared systems work similarly but use infrared light to transmit sound. A transmitter converts sound into a light signal that is beamed to receivers worn by listeners. The receivers decode the infrared signal and convert it back to sound.

For both FM and infrared systems, the receiver must be properly positioned relative to the transmitter or the sound quality will be poor. People with T-coils in their hearing aids or cochlear implants can connect to both FM and infrared systems via a neck loop.

CAPTION READERS FOR THEATERS

Shari's favorite theater-going experience of all time was seeing the Broadway production of *Hamilton* with captions. The speed of the dialogue and the intricacy of the lyrics would have been hard to follow without them. Any time she missed something, she glanced away from the action to the screen at the side of the stage to fill in the blanks. She caught every word!

Captioning devices are also available at the movies. A typical movie theater caption device has a display attached to an adjustable support arm that fits into a seat's cup holder. The screen is small, but the captions are clear. Privacy visors prevent the light from bothering others while the bendable arm lets you position the captions in a spot that works for you. Some movie theaters offer captioned glasses that display the captions in front of you as you watch the movie.

Most large movie chains now offer caption devices for all shows. Go to the ticket counter or concession stand to borrow one and return it at the end of the movie. How well the devices are maintained varies, but previews and pre-show ads are sometimes captioned, which is a good way to test if your device is working ahead of the main event.

Glitches are still common, unfortunately, especially in multi-theater complexes. Gael was at a show with her husband and son, and as the movie started, she was pleased to see that the captions were working, which wasn't always the case. But after a minute or so, she realized that what she was reading did not match what was happening on the screen! In fact, she looked at her young son and was thankful he couldn't see the rather passionate dialogue. The caption reader had been set to the wrong theater, and it took a few minutes for the staff to reset the reader to the right show.

COMMUNICATION GAME CHANGERS
Transforming the Conversation

GAEL: We spent the previous section raving about the joys of hearing technology. But there are *big* gaps in what technology alone can do. In this part, we are still raving, but this time about the gap-filling communication strategies that don't require batteries or electricity. These strategies will help you take back control of your communication.

 SHARI: You may already be using some of these crucial non-technical tools, but perhaps not all the time or in every situation. In this section, we take a deeper dive into communication game changers such as the simple but powerful act of letting others know about your hearing loss.

 GAEL: We talk about how to stop bluffing—the number one bad habit of people with hearing loss. It's kind of our dark-and-dirty secret. When we bluff, we sabotage all the other good things we do, like speechreading, to improve our life with hearing loss.

 SHARI: And we introduce HEAR, a brilliant tool (if we do say so ourselves) that will help you identify, ask for, and implement the changes you need to optimize any listening situation.

12

DON'T HIDE, SELF-IDENTIFY!

HEARING LOSS IS often referred to as an "invisible" disability. Unless your hearing devices are highly evident, or you say "pardon" every two or three sentences, casual acquaintances may not suspect your hearing loss. And if you say to that, "Great, I don't want them to!" we suggest a reread of the MindShifts section.

> **MindShift**
> Being open about my hearing loss will help me communicate better. Trying to hide my hearing loss leads to misunderstandings.

You may think you have been successful—so far—in keeping your hearing loss a secret. But have you? It may be possible for milder losses. Yet for all degrees of hearing loss, there are little clues that make people wonder, *What's going on with that person?*

Some will suspect the truth. But the vague look on your face or that you keep slowing down the conversation for repeats might lead them to another conclusion—perhaps that you are unfocused, slow on the uptake, or simply uninterested.

Isn't it better that they know the truth?

One of the most important tools in your skill-sack is the ability to confidently self-identify as having hearing loss. By stating it upfront, clearly laying out your needs and what can be done to meet them, you take charge of communication.

Many people are uncomfortable revealing this personal detail, but if you don't ask for the assistance you need, you won't get it.

HOW DO YOU DESCRIBE YOURSELF?

Before Shari came out of her hearing loss closet, she referred to her hearing loss only when absolutely necessary, mumbling something like, "I am sorry, I don't hear well." This statement morphed to "I have hearing loss" or "I wear hearing aids," but as she grew more comfortable, she began asking more directly for what she needed: "I have hearing loss and am having trouble hearing you. Would you please speak a little louder or slower?" Occasionally, if she's aiming for more impact, she says, "I'm a little bit deaf." That seems to get people's attention.

Gael was never in a hearing loss closet. From childhood she followed the pattern set by her parents, which was to disclose her hearing loss, especially to the people who *need* to know, such as teachers, friends, coworkers, and basically anyone she wants to communicate with.

Self-identification is her mantra, even though she occasionally succumbs to bluffing, which doesn't always end well. For most of her life, Gael described herself as "hard of hearing," but she now prefers to say that she has hearing loss or that she is deaf because, audiologically, that's what she is. She may even say, "I use a hearing aid and a cochlear implant." In her writing, she uses the term *HoH*, an acronym for hard of hearing, because it's snappy and fun and used by many on social media posts. But say "I'm a HoH" out loud, and you'll understand why you should only use the term with people who get what you mean.

Your hearing loss label is a personal choice. The variety of terms currently in use relate to identity with a community, degree of deafness, language or modes of communication, and longtime social use. Some of the terms are interchangeable, but some are not.

Deaf people—with a capital D—identify with Deaf Culture and use a signed language as their main means of communication. The term *deaf*—with a lowercase d—is used in different ways. Some people are deaf and use a spoken language to communicate; they may also use the term *oral deaf*. Some people with mild or moderate losses refer to themselves as "a little deaf."

Other common descriptors are *hard of hearing, person with hearing loss*, and *HoH*. These usually indicate people with some degree of hearing loss who use spoken language supported by hearing technology and other strategies. Some people also use the term *hearing impaired*, but this has largely fallen out of favor. These days, more people are choosing to skip the controversy by simply referencing their technology, as in "I use a hearing aid" or "I have a cochlear implant."

The debate about labels has caused unnecessary stress and division for decades. Far more important than the label you choose is your decision to be open about your communication needs. Language often reflects society and culture, meaning that change is likely the only constant. How you refer to yourself may change over time as you become more comfortable discussing your hearing issues. No matter what identity or label you choose, *it will be the right one for you.*

EXPLAINING YOUR HEARING LOSS

Telling people that you have hearing loss is simply informing them of a fact. The label you use to describe yourself doesn't explain what you need them to do or why. Self-identification alone is not enough. You must also help people who have no personal experience with hearing loss to understand it better. Using one of the following explanations might help them appreciate why you need them to speak louder but not yell:

"Hearing loss is like playing *Wheel of Fortune.*" Imagine a game board from this popular game show. Some of the letters are filled in and others are blank. This picture captures how people with hearing loss hear words and sentences. We must mentally combine incomplete sounds with visual speechreading cues to create words and phrases that make sense in the context of the conversation. It takes a lot of brain power and can be exhausting.

"I don't have peripheral hearing." This statement perfectly describes that for people with hearing loss, hearing is not passive; it is an active process that takes concentration and effort. Hearing is not something done in the background while performing another activity—it *is* the activity. This explanation also demonstrates why it is important for someone to get your attention before speaking. Unless you are listening alertly, you are not going to hear them start to speak, and by the time you tune in, you'll have missed the starting words.

"I hear with my eyes." For people with hearing loss, hearing is both auditory and visual. Body language, lips moving, and facial expression are all important clues in deciphering sounds. A friend of Shari's tells people, "Don't speak until you see the whites of my eyes" as a clear and humorous way to ask them to face her and to make compliance with the request more likely. (See more about visual cues in Chapter 13.)

SELF-IDENTIFYING IN GROUPS

Group conversations are challenging because the conversation zips and zags back and forth, making it hard to keep up. Unless you let people in the group know how to communicate with you, discussions will quickly spin out of control. You'll become so disconnected that you might as well just start playing a game on your phone.

In group conversations, Gael notices that people sometimes, without realizing it, address comments to others, leaving her out because she takes "more work" or because they don't realize she has been left behind. (It certainly can't be because she's not intelligent or interesting!) She understands why this happens because she sometimes does the same thing by not addressing people who she knows will be hard for her to understand. A MindShift could smooth this difficult situation and help you to re-engage in the conversation.

> **MindShift**
> I deserve to hear and be heard. I deserve to participate.

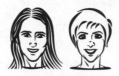

Far more important than
the label you choose to
describe your hearing
loss is your decision
to be open about your
communication needs.

At meetings or conferences, there are opportunities to disclose your hearing loss during introductions. When you say where you're from, and why you are there, you can add the juicy piece of information about your hearing loss, taking a moment to expand on what you need from others to be fully involved.

At Shari's most recent retreat, she began with the typical particulars but ended with: "Oh, and I just wanted to mention that I have hearing loss, so I will be positioning myself as close to the teacher as possible during the exercises." She gave a meaningful look in the teacher's direction to make sure she was listening. Then Shari said to the group, "If you speak to me and I don't answer, or if I look at you like you have two heads, please don't think I am rude—I probably just didn't hear you. Please try again."

Because she has to do it so often, Gael likes to shake up her introduction script. If someone says, "Oh, I'm sorry" when she mentions her hearing loss, Gael responds, "Don't be, I'm not." If someone asks what caused her deafness, she may reply, "I dunno. Just lucky, I guess." She explains that, yes, she reads lips, and when a person moves their head as they speak, she must also move hers to follow what they're saying. Gael also appreciates people who make unprompted efforts to communicate better, because changing how you interact isn't always easy.

When people know about your hearing loss, they are usually more understanding about swapping seats to give you a better view of the speaker or repeating something important that was said. They will understand that your mishears aren't because you are rude or inattentive. Being open also relieves the pressure of having to hear everything perfectly—and what a relief that is.

MAKE YOUR HEARING LOSS MORE VISIBLE

Rather than trying to hide their hearing loss, some people go the opposite way. Instead of using their hair to cover up their devices, people cut it short, putting their devices on vivid display. Isn't everyone wearing something on their head and in their ears these days?

Going one step further, people glam up their hearing aids and CIs with glitter, jewels, colorful stickers, and creative add-ons to make them more noticeable. Gael replaced the plastic security cord of her CI sound processor with a silver chain and ear cuff. Some people wear buttons or pins proclaiming their hearing loss with snappy sayings like *I Read Lips* or *Face Me, I Have Hearing Loss*. Some sew such messages onto face masks.

Several hearing loss websites offer cards that state your hearing loss. You can print them and carry them in your wallet or keep them in your car. These are useful when stopped by the police or in health emergencies.

13

SPEECHREADING BASICS

SPEECHREADING IS A fundamental communication strategy that people often employ without realizing it, whether or not they have hearing loss. The technique uses visual information to supplement what is heard, or sometimes to *completely* fill in what is not heard. You may not realize you are speechreading until a person turns away, obstructing their face from view.

"Gael, did I tell you Digby has fleas?" Gael's friend asked as he searched the fridge for snacks.

"That's a lot of fleas!" Gael replied.

Her friend looked back at her, confused.

"Digby's a huge dog, so that's a lot of fleas."

"Who said he has fleas?"

"You just did."

"I asked if you wanted a Diet Pepsi."

"Oh. Sure. Glad to hear Digby hasn't got fleas."

(She wasn't that glad. The hairy hound is the one that ate her thousand-dollar hearing aid the year before. Fleas would have been just desserts.)

This tale of fleas and Pepsi is the story of Gael's life. Like many people with hearing loss, she needs to see someone's face to understand them. She may hear that you are saying something, but she can't always distinguish the words. But look her in the eye, and she's yours forever.

People with hearing loss usually speechread naturally, without being aware of it, because everyone's brain, in its search for understanding, uses any sense it can to complete a task. But although speechreading may not need to be taught, the skill *can be* improved through some basic training and practice.

WHAT IS SPEECHREADING?

The terms *speechreading* and *lipreading* are both used to describe the process of using visual cues to understand speech.

Speechreading is a more complete term because when a person speaks, they use more than just their lips to convey a message. Your speechreading cues come from the movements of the lips, eyes, jaw, and tongue. You also use a person's facial expressions and body language, your knowledge of *context*—the subject being discussed—and what you actually *hear* to form a more complete idea of what is being said. It's a skill that comes naturally to some people, while others struggle with it.

The problem is that not all speech sounds are visible. In fact, fewer than 50 percent of speech sounds are visible on the lips, which is why you must observe other parts of the face and body for more clues.

Words are composed using a combination of lower-frequency vowels made with the voice-box, and higher-frequency consonants formed by movements of the breath, tongue, teeth, lips, and other facial muscles. Vowels give words their power, and consonants complete their meaning.

Many consonants are formed inside the mouth and can't be seen. To make things even more challenging, many consonants look the same on the lips. Consider the words *pat*, *bat*, and *mat*. Their sound is slightly different because they are formed differently, but they look the same and a speechreader may require the additional clues that come from context. Knowing whether the topic is pets, baseball, or flooring will clarify what word was said.

PRACTICE HELPS WITH COMPREHENSION

Why are some people better speechreaders than others? A major factor is how comfortable a person is at making eye contact: Eyeball-to-eyeball conversation is key to understanding. If you look around while conversing, or if you struggle with being attentive or patient, speechreading may be more difficult.

Speechreading success also depends on other factors, including your degree of hearing loss, whether you have high- or low-frequency loss, how well you can put all the clues together, and your visual acuity.

What's certain is that speechreading requires intense concentration. A great deal of energy goes into communication, which is why, at the end of the day, you may feel tired and experience eye strain. Part of any speechreading course involves learning how to rest your eyes and take frequent breaks to replenish the energy needed to connect.

Speechreading games are a fun way to practice this important skill and keep you nimble. Shari's children love "testing" her speechreading skills, making the games harder and harder until she is stumped—their favorite part! One night on vacation, they decided to try a lipreading-only dinner, with the kids mouthing their words and Shari replying with her voice.

A discussion of the sunset went smoothly. "What a beautiful sunset" and "Let's take a picture" were easy to speechread, especially since it was a stunning evening in paradise. Their thoughts about what to order were also simple since Shari could look down and scan the menu for reference. The conversation turned to movies and popular culture, and she sailed through talk about *Star Wars*, and even Matt Damon in his latest flick. But then they brought up another actor.

"Did they have an escape hatch?" Shari asked.

Her children giggled.

"Is someone walking down a lumber path?"

Peals of laughter. *Is "lumber path" even a thing?* Shari wondered.

"Are they bending in a cummerbund?"

Now her kids looked at her blankly. They hadn't been to many black-tie events.

Unfortunately, no clue could help because Shari had never heard of Benedict Cumberbatch! Eventually, they had to cheat and say his name out loud.

You can also practice speechreading by having someone read nursery rhymes and children's books with no voice or in a low voice. The sentences are short, rhythmic, and familiar, and you will score victories by recognizing well-known phrases on a person's lips. Having someone read a news story in the same manner is another good exercise. Note: The "reader" should use normal speech patterns at a moderate rate and non-exaggerated lip movements.

Speechreading exercises demonstrate how much energy we use in every communication situation. Not only are we using our ears to hear, but we also use our eyes to speechread and our brains to put it all together into something coherent. Even after we figure out what the person has said, we're not done, because then we need to reply! Speechreading is easier once you know the quirks and style of a person's speech. It takes time to develop that comfort with strangers unless they are very articulate.

There are many barriers to speechreading success—the biggest one, of course, is when the speaker's face isn't fully visible. Individual speaking styles—people who don't move their lips much, have whispery voices, or use rapid-fire speech—are also challenging. People may have accents that you find difficult to read because their mouths move in ways you're not used to seeing.

Gael is proud of her speechreading skill, but even the best speechreader has trouble following the conversation zipline at a dinner party. She has tried different tactics but hits a brick wall trying to convince a group of slightly inebriated people to speak one at a time or put their hands up when they wish to speak. You can get whiplash trying to keep up with person-to-person speechreading, so occasionally she resorts to thumping the table and saying, "What the hell are we talking about now?!"

It is difficult for people to change how they speak, even momentarily. And sometimes, certain people will simply be out of your speechreading grasp. But you can control speechreading barriers by asking speakers to:

- move their hands and other objects away from their face

- wait until they've finished chewing before speaking

- remove baseball caps or sunglasses that obscure the eyes

- turn their face so that it is better lit

Like any skill, speechreading ability comes with practice. Improve on your natural knack through online courses that can be purchased from hearing loss organizations. Play games like Shari's family does or use children's books. Encourage your partners to use normal speech rhythms when they mouth the words silently or in a low voice and to use full sentences rather than saying a few words at a time.

14

ADVOCATING FOR YOURSELF

THE ROLLING STONES tell us that we can't always get what we want. And we definitely won't get what we *don't ask for*! This is a fundamental lesson of hearing loss: You need to be assertive and specific about the help you need and just as clear about what you *don't* need.

When you advocate for yourself, you are also advocating for other people with hearing loss. By enlightening just one person about how to communicate with you, you create a ripple effect of awareness. Every one of your interactions—whether asking a restaurant manager to lower the volume of the music or requesting a caption reader at the movie theater—becomes a catalyst for broader and universal understanding of hearing loss issues.

> **MindShift**
> It is my right to ask for and receive equal access. When I advocate for myself, I am also creating change that benefits others.

ANTICIPATE BARRIERS

Wouldn't it be nice to walk into any social event, business meeting, entertainment venue, or other situation with the confidence that you will be able to hear well?

With hearing loss, this is not always a realistic expectation. Experiencing anticipatory anxiety—that feeling of fear or dread when you know you won't be able to hear very well at an event—is common. Some situations may seem so overwhelming that you decide to just stay home. Opting out is easier than struggling to hear in a noisy restaurant. It's less frustrating than trying to understand what the stage actors are saying. And it's certainly less emotionally taxing than hanging out with friends who should understand your needs but forget them in the organic flow of conversation.

But if you are tired of missing out on the fun, you *can* do something about it!

When you plan ahead, you can look forward to an event rather than dread it. By anticipating communication barriers, you can figure out ways to beat them. Would a different restaurant work better? Does the museum or theater have assistive listening systems? Is it time to try that microphone that brings voices into your hearing device?

Shari's family follows a ritual whenever they dine at a restaurant. First they make sure they are happy with the table—hopefully, it is in the quiet location they requested when they made the reservation. At the table, Shari chooses the seat that works best for her, ideally in a corner or with her back to a wall to limit background noise behind her. Then she arranges everyone else, situating the person who is hardest for her to hear diagonally across from her to aid with lipreading and to make sure that they will always be turned towards her when they speak. The person she hears the best sits next to her because she doesn't need to see them to hear them. *Then* they look at the menu.

To pick her most advantageous spot, Gael sometimes waits until everyone is seated, and then she rearranges people. This is primarily to assess and create the best possible communication flow, but watching the kerfuffle of people shuffling and sliding into other seats is also fun.

Take the following steps to deal with common listening challenges before you even arrive:

Whenever possible, be the one to pick the get-together location. You may already have a go-to list of restaurants, bars, or cafes that allow a decent conversation. Look for carpeting, lower ceilings (especially those with acoustic tiles), and soft surfaces like tablecloths and cushioned seats that absorb sound, making it easier to hear.

Do your research. Consult the website of an event or venue before visiting to determine what you need and what hearing assistance is available for the best experience.

Request accommodations well in advance. The more time you give a place to prepare for your visit, the more likely it is to be successful. At smaller venues, you might be the first person to ask for CART (see page 108) or other accommodations. Expect to educate staff about your needs and the options available to them. You may need to follow up several times to make sure they get things right.

Pack your tech tools. Some venues are less prepared to handle communication barriers, but this doesn't mean you can't enjoy your visit. Instead, you may need to bring your own assistive listening devices or apps to improve access.

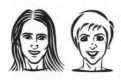

When you advocate for yourself, you are also advocating for other people with hearing loss.

FIGURE OUT WHAT YOU NEED AND ASK FOR IT

Hearing loss can be confusing to people who don't have it. Just when they think they've got you figured out, you change it up. One time, you ask them to *speak up!* The next time, you say *not so loud!* You likely don't need the same communication assistance all the time, but other people have no way of predicting this. You can't expect them to know exactly *how* you are perceiving sound at any given moment, because it *changes*.

When you are tired or anxious, you likely don't focus as well as you need to, so your hearing may seem to "drop." Background noise doesn't always interfere with the ability of hearing people to understand speech. But for you, that same noise can make the difference between understanding and not.

People won't automatically adjust to your fluctuating hearing needs. So your job is to articulate them as often as required—which is usually very often—and to feel comfortable doing so. For example, you might need:

- changes in speech—clearer, slower, louder, and so on

- clear sightlines to the speaker, especially to their face

- minimal background noise, which can overshadow speech

- good lighting for speechreading

- for others to use a microphone

- for people to speak one at a time

Staff at museums and other venues sometimes get confused about accommodations, so make your requests as specific as possible. Detail the type of technology you require, including whether you use a telecoil or Bluetooth to connect your hearing aids to other devices.

Many places think of sign language interpreters when people with hearing loss ask for accommodation. For the Deaf community this is vital communication access, but most people with hearing loss don't use or understand sign language. When requesting accommodations at public places, hospitals, museums, and other similar places, let them know that you do not sign.

TELL PEOPLE WHAT YOU DON'T NEED

Shari attended a fundraiser for a hearing loss charity many years ago. Cyndi Lauper performed. At first, Shari was surprised at the choice of a pop singer. Wouldn't the music be too loud? Was that the kind of message a hearing loss organization should send? Her worry was misplaced; the volume level was safe, and Lauper put on a great show.

The pop star, however, seemed mystified by the reduced volume level, as though she didn't know why the organizers had asked her to play the music so quietly. Considering her audience—most of whom had hearing loss—Lauper probably thought they would need her to play louder! Lauper wondered aloud "Why not turn up the volume?" which, delivered in Lauper's characteristic accent and style, made Shari laugh out loud. But the memory has stayed with her because the story reveals a common myth—that making something louder solves all hearing problems. With hearing loss, louder is not always better.

For Gael, louder is better only when she needs someone to speak up. But what she *doesn't* need is over-enunciation of words when she asks for a repeat—it is mildly patronizing, and distorted lips are difficult to speechread. Or being directed to "Tell me what I just said?" That's just humiliating, especially if you can't repeat the words, and there are better ways to ensure that someone is following. (Thank you, end of rant!)

Because hearing loss is so misunderstood by those who don't have it, people may attempt to help you hear better, but their efforts are often counterproductive. They might shout at you. Talking too slowly is also counterproductive because it causes lip distortion. Clarity of the sound is far more important, as well as context clues. Your conversation partners need to understand these important speech issues.

ASK FOR REPEATS

Saying "pardon" or "could you please repeat that" can feel uncomfortable—*I don't want to interrupt the flow of the conversation. Maybe I will catch on in a minute. Why bother?* You might prefer *not* to have to ask someone to repeat what they just finished saying, but it is an inevitable part of the hearing loss life and doing it is important.

If you don't ask for clarification or repeats when you need them, you risk becoming isolated and sliding into the bluff zone. The people in your life become accustomed to repeating themselves, just like Gael's Hearing Husband. He says something and then immediately repeats it, sometimes even a third time. (She finds this irritating, especially if she *did* catch it the first time.)

It may feel awkward or embarrassing at first to ask others to repeat themselves, but with practice comes confidence—and a thicker skin to deal with less than cooperative responses, especially from people who don't know you very well.

When you ask for a repeat once, people usually give it graciously. Ask twice, and they repeat it with concern. Ask a third time, and you are likely to draw impatience, a frown, and a little eyeball rolling. And the dreaded "oh never mind, it's not important" can happen at any stage.

How should you ask? The standard phrases are usually all that are required: *What? Pardon? Can you repeat that?*

But sometimes you don't even need to use words—a hand cupped behind the ear is the universal sign for "I can't hear you." And with people you know well, a raised eyebrow or even a quick lift of your chin with an enquiring look might be enough to tell them that you didn't catch what they just said.

Sometimes, you don't need a full repeat—just a clarification of a word or phrase. Or you may want to make sure you heard something correctly. You can do this by repeating what you think you heard, so your conversation partner only needs to repeat the part you missed. Often a repeat works better when it is rephrased.

DON'T ACCEPT DISMISSAL

It happens sometimes. A friend or colleague is telling a funny story or explaining an event that happened, and at some point Shari asks, "What did you say?" She got the beginning but missed a segment along the way and needs clarification. The speaker pauses, as if to think about the question, and replies, "Never mind." Usually, this is accompanied by a dismissive wave of the hand or shake of the head or both. Ouch, that hurts.

Never mind is a dismissal and an insult. So are *forget it*, *it's not important*, and *don't worry about it*. These responses say that the listener is not important enough to the speaker for them to repeat themselves. When people with hearing loss hear this, we may react angrily, or we may simply tune out. It may also be the end of our interactions with that person.

When it is perceived as a rejection, this dismissal of hearing loss needs can also lead to social isolation. Giving up the effort to assert your needs may seem better than being publicly dismissed or shamed but could also start a downward emotional spiral. A more effective approach is to help people understand how hurtful their statement is to you.

If someone tells you "never mind," respond with, "Please, I really would like to hear what you have to say." Saying no to that is a challenge, and your assertiveness will show that dismissal is not an option. Quite often, the person honestly believes that their original comment is not worth repeating, but you want to be the judge of that.

THEY AREN'T MIND READERS

You know the hearing loss drill so well that you expect others to know it, too. This thinking is an easy trap of frustration to fall into.

"I can't hear people when they are facing away from me," Shari called out from the rear on a recent family hike. Nobody answered.

"I can't hear what you are saying if I am in the back," she said, a bit louder this time.

"Okay," one of them replied, but nobody moved. She was starting to get annoyed.

They stopped at an outlook, and before they continued on Shari said, "I want to be second in the line so I can hear," and immediately, the sea parted.

"Why didn't we do this in the first place?" she wondered aloud.

"You didn't use your words, Mom," her son told her.

"I did, but nobody listened."

Whenever they were upset as children, she would ask them to use their words to explain the problem instead of crying or whining. That way they could work together to find a solution. Now that they are teenagers, they enjoy throwing her words of wisdom back at her.

"You didn't use your words," he repeated.

He was right. Shari had used words, but only to point out the obvious—if she was in the back, she would not hear well, if at all. She had not been specific about what she needed. She was relying on them to read her mind rather than making explicit requests. She was being passive, rather than assertive, complaining rather than advocating for her needs.

You may find that you're requiring people to anticipate your needs or to read between the lines of your statements and know what to do to accommodate your hearing loss. This is not always fair. As people with hearing loss, our responsibility is to be straightforward and up front with our requests—the more specific the better. Only then can we expect others to act the way we need.

15

NO BLUFFING!

IF THERE'S ONE habit shared by almost every person with hearing loss, it's pretending that they understand what's being said—when they don't. But when you bluff, you are *not* advocating for yourself.

When Gael was in her twenties, she was dating a Nice Guy, and they went for a walk along the beach one night. This was not an ideal date setting for someone like Gael, who needs either a flashlight or the ability to walk backward without falling over logs to speechread someone walking with her, especially in the dark.

The Nice Guy asked Gael something, and she didn't catch it. It was just one more hearing frustration, and she knew she would probably have to ask him to repeat himself more than once. Since it sounded like a question requiring either a yes or a no answer, she picked one—she figured it was fifty-fifty that she'd get it right—and so she said *no*.

By his reaction, she knew her answer was unexpected. And somehow wrong. But there was no turning back (she wasn't skilled in hearing loss communication best practices back then) and she repeated herself. No.

Fizzle-fizzle, end of relationship—no more Mr. Nice Guy—and she still has no idea what he asked her. But she can guess: "I like you, Gael, do you like me?"

"No."

"Oh. Uh, you don't want to go out anymore?"

"No."

So, if you're looking for relationship advice, Gael can recommend bluffing as the perfect way to poke a sharp stick in the eye of a relationship. She kicked herself for a long time afterwards because, in spite of not remembering his name now, she liked that guy. Her stubborn bluffing sabotaged what may have been a good thing.

Bluffing, faking, and *passing* are all words that describe what happens when you fall into a communication black hole. Some people lapse occasionally, but others make it a frequent, almost chronic, bad habit.

Some people are so skilled at bluffing that no one would ever guess they are doing it. But is that a good thing? If you make it all the way through a conversation without getting caught out, what's the benefit? You have no idea what just went down; what if it was something important? Did you agree to host a party? Go on a date? Worship a different deity?

What's worse is recognizing some serious gaps in your comprehension of a conversation and then feeling embarrassed because you must now have *this* conversation:

"Look, friend, I really didn't catch what was said back there."

"Which part didn't you catch, the ending bit?"

"Uh, the beginning bit. Also, the middle. And the ending."

"Seriously? Why didn't you say something?"

There are many reasons why we bluff, but no good reason why we should, and many good reasons why we definitely should not. This so-called skill seldom has positive results and often backfires. Some spectacular bluffs can haunt us for years. *Why did I have to laugh when she was telling us the sad news about her pet? What if he was asking me to marry him that night and I said no? Why didn't I just ask for a repeat?*

WHY DO YOU BLUFF?

Bluffing isn't entirely due to stubbornness or impatience. The reasons for bluffing are individual and complex, dictated by your personality, type and degree of hearing loss, and understanding and acceptance of the loss. Sometimes you may not even realize that you are bluffing, at least not right away. But when you become aware, why do you keep on doing it?

The triggers for bluffing are similar to those for any challenging interaction: a noisy, poorly lit room; people whose speech characteristics make them difficult to hear or speechread; or group conversations that spin away out of your control.

But the main reasons for bluffing—and why you might keep on bluffing even when you're aware of doing it—are more personal:

- lack of assertiveness and communication skills

- uncertainty about how to stop bluffing and not lose face with others

- the desire to hide your hearing loss, both generally and in specific listening situations

- fear of appearing inadequate or slow

- misplaced politeness (you don't want to annoy or interrupt others)

- it's become a bad habit

- weariness of asking for repeats

- exhaustion from trying to keep up

- deliberately choosing to "sit this one out"

- and more...

Some people with hearing loss have perfected their bluffing game. They have a number of ways to bluff: using the silent treatment, repeating an occasional word they *do* hear to give the false impression of being involved, and copying reactions from other people.

But rather than becoming a better bluffer, why not become a better communicator?

16

ADOPTING "HEAR"

H OW *DO YOU* become a better communicator? We wrestled with this question for years. When we began this book, we discovered that at some point, we had both independently adopted the same simple steps to evaluate and improve any listening situation. This realization was a major communication game changer.

We call these steps HEAR. This communication checklist, the mother of all Hearing Hacks, is a quick and effective process to determine what needs to change in any communication situation and how to make it happen. With practice, HEAR will become second nature.

Step	Actions
Hearing check	Can I understand what my communication partner is saying?
Evaluate	What do I need to improve the listening environment? More light? Less noise? Louder speech? Slower speech? A different seat?
Articulate	Ask for what you need for better communication. Your communication partners will also benefit.
Revise and remind	Adjust as needed. Remind conversation partners if they fall back into old speech habits.

H: HEARING CHECK

Use this in any and every listening situation. Ask yourself, *Can I understand what others are saying?* Adjusting to a new setting may take some time, but if after a couple of minutes of listening the answer is anything less than a solid yes, something needs to change.

E: EVALUATE

What would improve the situation?

Start by assessing the **environment**. Is loud music playing? Does the lighting need to be brighter? Would a different area of the room be quieter and more conducive to conversation? Can you add more soft surfaces like pillows or a tablecloth to absorb sound? Will a different seating arrangement prevent you from facing into bright light or allow you to see the faces of the other speakers? Can you sit in a corner or against a wall to minimize background noise?

Evaluate your **conversation partners**. Are they speaking too softly or quickly? Are they covering their mouths or turning away from you when they speak? Are people talking over one another? Are some of your companions harder for you to hear? The more you use this assessment, the more ingrained and intuitive—and the faster—it will become.

Consider your available **technology** tools. Would a speech-to-text app or a sound amplifier app help you follow the dialogue? Is there a better setting on your hearing aid for this type of situation, or can you use your remote microphone to bring the important speech sounds into your devices? If so, use them!

A: ARTICULATE

This is often the hardest part—telling others what you need. Do not skip this step. Recite a MindShift if you need to.

> **MindShift**
> I deserve to hear and be heard. I deserve to participate.

To fix environmental problems, you will need to speak to someone at the venue or your host at a private home. If you are reluctant to ask for the lights to be turned up or the noise turned down, don't forget that you are a guest who deserves to at least have your requests heard.

Learning to do this *assertively* rather than aggressively ensures a better result. Aggressive behavior indicates that your needs are more important than anyone else's, while being assertive means you're standing up for yourself, but with respect for others as well.

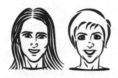

If you are comfortable with your hearing loss, others will be, too.

Even when you think you are asking in a nice way, your facial expressions and body language may be saying something different. For example, when you are frustrated or concerned about a potential problem, you may frown and show tension. People with hearing loss must concentrate *so* hard to hear—especially in a difficult environment. You may be wearing a super frown! Even when you are not angry, you may look like you are, and this can be off-putting. So, before you ask, do a mental face check to smooth out a possible frown. There's an old saying that "you catch more flies with honey than with vinegar."

Regardless of your facial expression, if your request is met with resistance, ask for suggestions from your host or the venue to improve the situation. Or suggest an alternative yourself. Persistence may be required, but one thing is for sure—they are more likely to honor your requests if your manner is gently persuasive.

A brave group of four people with hearing issues, including Shari, went out to dinner one Friday night. Between them, they had six hearing aids, two cochlear implants, and one very handy remote microphone which would help them enjoy great conversation—but only once they found the right seat.

When they arrived at the restaurant, they asked for a table in a quiet location, explaining that most of them had hearing issues. They had forgotten to note this when they made the original reservation, which was a mistake. Despite this oversight, the hostess said she had a quiet spot for them, and they were thrilled. Until she sat them in the center of a noisy room. As they took their seats, they knew they were going to have a problem.

They explained their situation to the manager. After a moment's thought, he mentioned that the bar area had a table available. They were skeptical—bar areas are notoriously loud—but it turned out to be much better. After moving to the bar, they enjoyed the quieter surroundings, the food, drink, and each other's company. They couldn't hear perfectly, but the conversation flowed more easily than it would have in the first location.

They also learned an important lesson in self-advocacy. Despite the disappointment of the first table, no one got upset, raised their voice, or caused a scene. By politely asking a second time for an accommodation, they found someone who could help and a solution that worked well.

When the problem is not your environment but how your conversation partners speak, be clear about what you need them to do. Instead of "I hope you don't mind, but could we speak one at a time, maybe?" or "I keep asking you this—you always forget about me," try this: "Hey guys, let's slow it down a bit so I can catch what everyone is saying."

Hopefully, over time and with frequent reminders, your friends and family will adopt the drill. But strangers will still require your well-honed hearing loss script: "I have hearing loss and am having trouble hearing you. Could you please speak one at a time and a bit slower, move your hand away from your face, and stop chewing and swallow before speaking?" Or just articulate the piece that you really need, such as, "Let's move to a quieter table."

If you are reluctant to ask a group of people to adjust their behavior just for you, remember that *everyone* benefits from a courteous, smooth-flowing conversation.

R: REVISE AND REMIND

Perhaps a musician arrives and the noise level picks up or the lights dim to create a more romantic ambiance. You may need to readjust the seating arrangement or employ a new assistive listening technology to combat a new obstacle. Reapply HEAR's steps when the listening situation changes.

Reminders are almost always required—they are a constant in the hearing loss life. Often, your conversation partners will comply with your communication requests, but after a while with no visible reminder, and because you *seem* to be understanding, they revert to their typical speech patterns. They may begin to speak over one another or mumble or start to speed talk again. It's time for another reminder.

Although you may expect strangers to forget to speak louder or keep their faces uncovered, it's frustrating when your family and friends forget what you need. This is hurtful. *They should know I can't hear them when they all talk at once!* A well-placed hand behind the ear might shift their awareness, but if a verbal reminder is necessary, offer it in a positive way. It makes your reminders more effective.

Have a little compassion! Sustaining an unaccustomed speech style is difficult. For example, someone with a naturally soft voice may be very uncomfortable in speaking louder because to their own ears, they are yelling.

> **MindShift**
> Communication improves with practice. I will forgive myself when I'm not perfect. I am grateful for the efforts of others, even when they're not perfect.

But don't give up on asking for what you need. Be persistent! If you can find the humor in your mishears, which *are* often hilarious, laugh about it. It helps other people feel better about the situation, making them even more amenable to repeating things in a way you can understand. If you are comfortable with your hearing loss, others will be, too.

17

COMMUNICATION BEST PRACTICES

HEAR IMPROVES ALMOST any listening situation. But while people with typical hearing often bear the bigger burden for behavior change (for example, in adjusting the pace and style of their speech), people with hearing loss must drive the process. It's the communication-is-a-two-way-street thing.

TIPS FOR YOUR CONVERSATION PARTNERS

Share the following ideas with the important people in your life so they understand their critical role in good communication:

Get your attention before speaking. When you have hearing loss, you don't necessarily realize a person has started speaking and may miss important context in the first few phrases. Ask your conversation partners to give you a heads-up before speaking so that you don't need to play catch-up.

Watch for comprehension. If they see you leaning towards them or looking confused, they can take it as a cue to slow down or speak louder. They can also check in with you to make sure you understood what they said before continuing to speak.

Provide context. Knowing the topic of conversation makes it easier for you to guess more accurately the words you don't hear. If you know the conversation is about clothing, predicting that "—oot" is *suit*, and not *fruit*, is easier.

Speak clearly. Shouting or speaking extra slowly will distort their lips, making speechreading more challenging. Maintaining a moderate pace at a normal volume will provide more processing time for you to understand what they are saying.

Provide an unobstructed view. Providing a clear sightline of their face and keeping their mouth free of obstructions is important. Speechreading is easier when you don't have to watch them chew their food as they speak. Ball caps and sunglasses shade or hide facial cues. Also, we can't hear around corners or through walls.

Match facial expressions and body language to words. Facial expressions and body language reinforce the emotions behind the words and are important visual cues for people who speechread.

Be aware of surroundings. Background noise is always a barrier. Turn off the AC or at least turn the fan down to low and don't play background music. Choose a quieter restaurant or request a corner booth. A quiet and well-lit spot always works best.

Take turns speaking. If there are multiple people in the conversation, they can speak one at a time and each speaker can face you when they talk. Truthfully, this is not easy to sustain, but it is a worthy goal.

Repeat or rephrase. They should be prepared to comply with requests for repeats. But if you do not get it the first or even second time, they can try rephrasing their thoughts, because different words might actually be easier for you to hear. They could also spell a word that is giving you a particularly hard time. Knowing the first few letters of a word may help you to connect the dots.

Keep a sense of humor. Hearing loss communication can cause frustration—that's a real and acceptable emotion. Encourage them to feel comfortable in laughing at the mishears and misunderstandings. As long as they understand that they are laughing *with* you and not *at* you, humor is one way to get through the challenge.

TIPS FOR YOU

Conversation is a back-and-forth activity. People will adjust their communication styles with you, but *you* need to accommodate them as well. The following are actions you can use to facilitate better communication:

Review the section above. All the tips apply to you, too. Sometimes you might be just as guilty of communication missteps as the hearing people in your life.

Learn to listen again. Those who have lived with hearing loss for some time before adopting hearing aids or other devices may have developed poor listening habits, such as tuning out, bluffing, and simply waiting for their turn to talk. If you have decided to hear and communicate better, you must be more mindful in conversations and attuned to other speakers. Otherwise, when you hit minor roadblocks, you may slide back into old habits.

Repeat bits that you do hear. Rather than ask for a full repeat, verbalize the part of the statement that you did hear. This will help the speaker better understand what to say again or rephrase.

Get enough rest. People with hearing loss often hear better in the morning after a good night of rest and relaxation for the brain. Schedule important conversations for early in the day so you can bring your strongest communication game to the meeting. If this is not possible, try to factor in rest time ahead of the event to recharge your listening batteries.

Be prepared. When you know what the conversation is going to be about, at meetings, for example, you will be better able to understand and participate. Knowing a movie's theme and plot makes it easier to follow. Understanding a new name (of a country or a celebrity or a neighbor, for example) is easier when you've already seen or heard it.

Remember your MindShifts. Maintaining a positive approach to communication will pay off in better relationships and just about every aspect of your life.

18

WHEN NOTHING ELSE WORKS

THE MUSIC WAS blaring. People were covering their ears. Shari had turned her hearing aids off but could still feel the bass reverberating through her body. How could anybody think this would be a good setting for a reunion? Most people were just trying to survive acoustically—shouting to one another to be heard or attempting to find a quieter spot for discussion. Some danced rather than attempting conversation or simply focused on eating in silence.

Shari was miserable. She couldn't effectively talk to anyone—speechreading can take you only so far—and she kept worrying whether the wall of noise was further damaging her hearing. She didn't want to be "anti-social" or miss the "fun," but she had to get out of there. When she fled the party, though, she was overwhelmed with guilt and self-loathing. *Why couldn't I figure out a way to make the situation work? Where were my self-advocacy skills? Why didn't I just ask someone to turn down the music?*

In time she realized she had done the right thing. Some situations are not worth the effort required to conquer them—and some just aren't possible to master. Even though it felt like defeat at the time, it was self-advocacy—of the most important kind.

Sometimes nothing you do seems to improve a challenging, even nightmarish, situation. What to do? You can bluff, smiling and nodding like a bobblehead figure. She knows she shouldn't, but sometimes, in the most difficult situations, this is Gael's fallback position, even now, as a strong anti-bluffing advocate. Sometimes she gives herself permission to "sit this one out" quietly, in her own mind, because the listening situation is taking more energy than she has. Other times she says, "Hey people. This just isn't working for me. Love you, bye!"

As much as you try to fix them, some situations are not conducive to good conversation, and despite all your MindShifts, technology, and communication game changers, you are not going to be able to communicate well. As long as this is the exception and not the rule, give yourself permission to retreat. Forgive yourself and vow to fight again another day.

RELATIONSHIPS AND SUPPORT NETWORKS

Bringing Your People with You

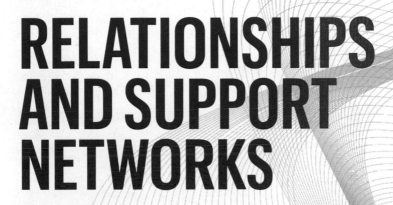

SHARI: When I think about the most frustrating aspects of my hearing loss, it always comes down to how it has impacted my relationships, such as the easy conversation with a loved one that now takes work or the friendship that faded because conversing was just too hard.

 GAEL: Regardless of the relationship type—partner, friend, colleague—there's a filtering process unique to people with hearing loss. Nice person? Check. Fun to be around? Check. Intelligent? Check. Then there's an extra question: Speak clearly? If it's not a check, then no matter how wonderful the other qualities are, the relationship is going to be challenging.

 SHARI: But sometimes we don't get to choose. Our family, children, or even our doctors or bosses may be hard for us to understand. We must find ways to take these important partners with us on our hearing loss journey.

 GAEL: In this part of the book, we share strategies for doing just that—ways to "make it work" at home, at the office, and everywhere in between—including the often overlooked but invaluable relationship in the life of anyone with hearing loss: the one with your hearing care professional.

19

THE IMPACT ON RELATIONSHIPS

EARING LOSS SLAMS its biggest fist into relationships—which are often the most valued part of a person's life. Whether your relationship is with a significant other, parents, children, friends, or business associates, or even just that nice person at the corner store, hearing loss can disrupt your communication, which is the glue that binds us together.

When your hearing changes, your behavior often changes, too. It's common to start avoiding once-loved activities—from parties to concerts to playing cards—because of debilitating background noise or difficult group interactions. And if you previously enjoyed these activities with a partner or close friends, the changes may strain the relationship. You might become frustrated at not being able to participate as fully as before, while your companion may resent your withdrawal. Both sides may feel powerless if neither of you knows how to improve the situation.

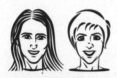

Dealing with hearing loss is like trying to catch a fish with your bare hands. Just when you think you've got it, off it wriggles in a different direction.

Support and understanding are a two-way street—just like good communication. There is a learning curve as both sides adapt. You must share your emotional struggles with your loved ones, and you must try to understand their frustrations.

Shari's father's hearing loss was an unmentionable topic, which made it almost impossible for his family to know how to help him when he was struggling. If he had been able to share his needs, the family might have stayed closer.

Dealing with hearing loss is like trying to catch a fish with your bare hands. Just when you think you've got it, off it wriggles in a different direction. Every listening situation is different, even if it seems the same. Some days you just hear better and don't require anything from others. Some days you need modifications.

Fluctuating needs can be confusing to communication partners who may commit blunders because they can't always perceive your current ability to hear. What worked yesterday might not work today. You may be tired and unable to focus on conversing, or the background noise may be different. And there's also the simple possibility that they, in that moment, simply forget your needs. They are subject to the same negative influences on good communication as you are: fatigue, impatience, or self-absorption in that moment. But there's more to it.

PEOPLE COMMUNICATE WITH EMOTIONS

Words are just the tip of the communication iceberg. The emotional tone of what you communicate to others is conveyed by your facial expressions, body language, eye contact, and tone of voice—which are the same informational cues you use when speechreading. But sometimes this unspoken information and the words you say send mixed messages. An example is the famous hearing loss frown.

When Gael was growing up, her mother would often say, "Smile, Gael!" This confused her because she didn't realize that she *wasn't* smiling, but she would humor her mother and flash a smile. Only as an adult, seeing videos of herself, did Gael realize her default face wears a frown—sometimes a fierce one! She swears it's not because she's grumpy, but a lifetime of intense focus on what's being spoken has carved a permanent groove between her eyes that could be easy to misunderstand. She has to consciously remind herself to smooth out those frown-grooves.

Another communication issue is that people with typical hearing don't realize how well they hear. They immediately register a noise as a cough, a bell, a door slam. When they hear words, no matter how poorly expressed, they *understand* them, and—get this— they even know where the sound is coming from! Everything that your average person with hearing loss *can't* do. We must listen with intention and effort, but for them the act of hearing is automatic.

When your partner or parent or child or friend forgets to face you, or isn't being attentive enough to your needs, your irritation may flare. You've told them a million times not to call you from another room! You've asked them not to talk-and-walk-away! You shouldn't have to remind them every time to face you!

But hearing people get irritated, too.

They've asked you not to bluff (because they can tell you're doing it). They've repeatedly hinted that you should visit the HCP again because something has changed with your hearing or devices. They've asked you to suggest ways to fix the listening environment— because you're the best judge of what works! And they may be hurt by your angry reactions when they make a mistake. You may need a MindShift.

> **MindShift**
> My hearing loss impacts my family and friends, too. We will learn how to be better communicators together.

WHY YOU NEED SUPPORT NETWORKS

Hearing loss is not a solo dance. It's more like a tango for two or a folk dance for many. It impacts everyone you communicate or regularly interact with. All of them are potential members of your hearing loss support team.

And you do need support.

But there's a difference between needing help and feeling helpless. People with hearing loss are *not helpless*, but good two-way communication requires the support of others. Even if you use hearing aids and other devices, effective conversations also require the willingness and ability of others to meet your needs.

A support network doesn't mean that people just cheer you on and listen to your emotional rants. They also offer tough love and tell you truthfully how you are doing. Members of your support team can help you adjust to new communication realities, because they must learn and develop comfort with the same things, at the same time.

Your support network may start to form well before your first visit to your HCP, with family and friends encouraging you to seek professional assistance when they see you struggling to hear. As your hearing loss journey progresses, that network will expand to include a trusted hearing care professional—one who understands your needs and helps you meet them.

You will also benefit from connecting to hearing loss peers who understand what you are experiencing. Even just one other person with hearing loss can make you feel less alone in your struggles, and most people are generous in sharing tips, tricks, and life hacks to smooth out your hearing loss journey.

When Gael was pregnant, she worried that her hearing loss might affect her ability to keep her baby safe. But in yet another world-changing moment, she met a young mom with hearing loss whose words of experience and encouragement assured her she could do it and her baby would be fine. The woman, now a lifelong friend, not only calmed Gael's nerves but also guided her to a new life as a hearing loss advocate.

When you tap into these sources of support, you create a solid, multi-block foundation for navigating the emotional and physical aspects of your hearing loss.

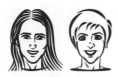

There's a difference between needing help and feeling helpless. People with hearing loss are *not helpless*; but to communicate better, they need the support of others.

20

FAMILY SUPPORT

THE STIGMA SHARI'S father felt about his hearing loss kept him from getting the help that he needed. When Shari started her own family, she knew she had to take a completely opposite tack. She talks about her hearing loss all the time—maybe too much for their liking—but they certainly know when she is struggling to hear and have become expert in helping her apply HEAR (hearing check, evaluate, articulate, revise and remind) in various settings. It's not always perfect. Their behavior still disappoints her sometimes, but she knows they have her back and are trying their best—and she can't imagine taking on the challenges of living with hearing loss without their tactical as well as emotional support.

When you have hearing loss, your family has it, too. It just affects them in different ways. And because you probably spend a lot of time with family (however you define family), recruiting them to your support team is crucial.

It starts with creating an open dialogue about your hearing loss.

TALKING TO FAMILY

Hearing loss is hard to describe and takes time to understand. And family members aren't always the most patient with those they love. The sad fact is that many families don't do anything to support their child or adult family member with hearing loss, and the repercussions of this can last a lifetime.

If your hearing loss is not acknowledged by a parent, you may grow up thinking you are stupid and you may not understand why you struggle. When you finally learn the truth, it can be a difficult, painful shock on many levels. If this is your situation and your family is still not open to discussing your hearing loss, reach out for other resources including counseling and peer support. If you haven't begun moving forward already, make this moment—now, as you're reading this book—your new starting point.

Or you may feel like your family recognizes your hearing loss, but they are not interested in helping you with it. They may say, "You hear what you want to hear" or ask you to turn up your hearing aids. This may come from a lack of understanding—but the result is a hurtful dismissal of your struggles. Their attitude may be that if you can't keep up, you deserve to be left behind. And some people simply don't see why *they* should have to change to accommodate another person's issue.

If you want better family communication, you have to help them understand, and they have to listen. When the reality of hearing loss is clearly explained and the *will* to communicate exists, partners, parents, and children can come closer together as they deal with an issue affecting them all.

But how do you do that?

After a family meeting about my hearing loss, I noticed an immediate difference in their behavior. I hope it sticks.

RECRUITING YOUR FAMILY TO YOUR TEAM

One Saturday morning, Shari's husband called the family together. "We need to talk about your mother's hearing loss," he said, "and how we can do a better job to help her hear." At first, the kids were annoyed with this. "We talk about this all the time," they said. "We know what to do."

"But we need to do better," he declared. "She is an important part of this family, and we love her. It is our responsibility to help her hear." Shari was blinking back tears.

Truth be told, the conversation was a bit repetitive of others they'd had before, but the formality of it was different. More serious and more memorable. Shari noticed an immediate shift in her family's behavior.

Getting people on your hearing loss team takes time and repeated effort. Think of it like a coach training a sports team. Here are some ideas to help build your family team:

Use an exercise for a glimpse into your hearing difficulties. Have your family wear earplugs at the next family dinner or on a commute to school or the office—any activity that normally requires them to listen and talk. This won't be a completely accurate experience since earplugs don't mimic the distortion that comes with hearing loss, and they'll still have the assurance that, sometime soon, they'll be able to take out the earplugs and return to their stellar hearing. But it will give them an idea. After the experiment, discuss what they experienced and the frustrations they encountered. This exercise may lead them to at least one important MindShift of their own.

Share your emotions about your hearing loss. Acknowledge your anger and sadness—they can see it anyway. Keeping it inside may give the impression that you have it under control or that you don't want to talk about it. The more you share, the easier it will be for them to provide the support that you need. Vulnerability is a path to true partnership. When you share what scares you most, it will help them be brave and share their feelings, too.

Normalize your hearing loss. Talking about your hearing loss breaks down any stigma attached to it. Make your hearing loss a normal part of the family dynamic, just like a child's *Star Wars* obsession or a severe allergy. If the family wants to go to the movies, find a theater with closed captioning devices. A restaurant choice should depend on how loud it is and if you can reserve a quiet table in the back. The more hearing loss is treated as normal, the more normal it becomes.

Teach them communication best practices. They may not know how to help you communicate well. Explain the steps involved in HEAR (hearing check, evaluate, articulate, revise and remind) and educate them about the communication best practices found on page 155. These practices may not be obvious to people with little experience with hearing loss, but small changes in behavior can turn a frustrating conversation into a more satisfying one for both sides. The more your family knows, the more they can help.

Involve your family in the fun part of hearing loss. *The fun part?* Ask them to help you experiment with new technologies like apps and assistive listening devices. Your family members are perfect guinea pigs, and it can be an adventure, especially with kids or grandkids who may think these gadgets are cool.

Ask them to partner with you in self-advocacy. When your family is familiar with your needs and with HEAR, they can help you resolve problems much faster. They can help you evaluate any hearing situation and to articulate your needs. When your family asks the restaurant manager to lower the music or collects the caption reader at the movies for you, you feel the warmth of their strong support.

BRING YOUR FAMILY TO AN APPOINTMENT

When Shari first began acknowledging her hearing loss, she brought her husband with her to audiologist appointments. His emotional support was helpful, especially as she was still overcoming significant self-imposed stigma about wearing hearing aids. But once she was fitted with her first pair, he stopped coming. Perhaps that was a mistake. Two sets of ears are always better than one.

Consider taking your family to your next appointment with your HCP. Seeing data—including your audiogram and other test results—and comparing them to those of a person with typical hearing is an eye-opener! Your HCP unemotionally and expertly explaining the data to your family will boost the significance of your results. It may also tangibly frame your hearing loss, making it easier for them to grasp your issues.

With a more nuanced understanding of how your hearing loss manifests itself in everyday life, they may take it more seriously and be less likely to unfairly blame you when communication breaks down. Ask your HCP to share tips for better conversations. Although these may be the same requests you make daily—face me, slow down, and so on—they will be more powerful if an expert confirms them.

Your family can also share their perspective on which communication situations are most challenging for you. This provides an outside take on how well you manipulate your devices. When the Hearing Husband joined Gael for an appointment to discuss her tinnitus, she was stunned to hear him describe the emotional effect it had on her and on their life together. He had never articulated this before, at least not in front of her, and as he did, he teared up. It was a stunning demonstration of how deeply our hearing issues affect those closest to us.

The more your HCP knows about your life, the better they can tailor their recommendations to your specific needs. Appointments that include family members provide useful information from a different point of view. Like any important medical consultation, two brains are better than one in catching important details.

FORGIVE THEM WHEN THEY DISAPPOINT YOU

At times, our friends and family will disappoint us. At the end of a wonderful day of vacation, Shari and her family headed to the hotel bar balcony to relax. The space was quiet, so they dropped their voices to match the ambience. Shari knew this was a natural reaction, but because she couldn't hear them, she asked her family to speak louder. They didn't need to shout, but simply talk at a normal volume, as the other people on the balcony were doing.

But her family couldn't do it. Or wouldn't do it. They glanced around with embarrassment as they continued to speak and laugh with one another in quiet voices. They seemed more concerned about not disturbing others on the balcony than about including Shari in the conversation. When the balcony got busier and noisier, their voices returned to normal. But Shari was still hurt by their dismissive behavior. Then she remembered: *My family is usually very supportive. I should probably give them a pass once in a while.* Nobody can expect perfection, but it still didn't feel good.

When your friends and family forget to use—or choose not to use—communication best practices, it can be hurtful. These are the people who should know *best* what you need. But consider that you spend most of your meaningful time with these people and so there are more opportunities for them to slip up. Communication boo-boos are going to happen—a lot—and making a big fuss every time might be counterproductive. Save your energy for the big stuff and try to focus on what they are doing right, accepting that you will need to remind them over and over again.

MindShift
Communication improves with practice. I forgive myself when I'm not perfect. I am grateful for the efforts of others, even when they're not perfect.

It might also help to share resources (such as this book) with them. Difficult and potentially emotional information is often digested better when it comes from a neutral party.

21

ROMANTIC RELATIONSHIPS

ALL THE RULES change when it comes to intimate relationships. Communication strategies that work reasonably well with your parents, children, or other family members somehow don't work the same way. Your best friend might repeatedly forget to face you before starting to talk and you just roll your eyes and remind her again. But when your romantic partner does the same thing, you blow up or retreat into icy silence.

More than any other type of relationship, romantic liaisons thrive on good communication. When hearing loss enters the equation, strategies need to be redesigned and *practiced* because there is a lot more at stake. And some extra creativity is required when hearing loss enters the bedroom.

The work starts on the very first date.

DATING: IS HEARING LOSS A THIRD WHEEL?

A hearing loss friend once told Shari that one of his major criteria for dating someone was the sound of his date's voice. Could he hear her easily or not? If he couldn't, there was no second date. That may sound harsh, but it's smart; why pursue a relationship with someone whose natural voice is impossible to understand?

Gael's must-haves in someone to date (or spend her life with) went beyond the standard handsome, funny, and smart; the list included lips big enough to speechread and a voice deep enough to hear. She couldn't hide her hearing loss from the man who ultimately became her life partner because they met at work and he already knew about it. Her hearing loss didn't bother him, and his speechread-able face mattered a lot to her. So they got married.

But sometimes knowing when to disclose hearing loss to a potential partner is difficult. Do you say your name and pop out with: "I have hearing loss, and this is what I need you to do if we're going to have a good conversation and possibly a great relationship?"

Perhaps you don't want to disclose your hearing loss right away, worrying, *Maybe my date will be turned off by it.* The plan might be to "wait and see how this goes." But *this* is how it usually goes: You get caught in an embarrassing situation. Perhaps you've said "pardon" three times—forcing you to admit your hearing loss, only to find that it wasn't a secret because you had already answered a question inappropriately.

"Would you like something to drink?"

"Why, thank you—my mother gave it to me."

Also, your hearing aid might not be as invisible as you think.

The same question applies to online dating: At what point do you disclose? The choice is yours. You might want to state it upfront in a profile, at first connection, after a few get-to-know-you texts, or put it off until the first face-to-face meeting.

Regardless of how you meet someone, you can avoid the awkward stuff by being direct. Hearing loss is not a turnoff unless you make it one. If the "whole package of you" is something this other person finds attractive, don't muck it up by trying to hide an important part of that package.

> **MindShift**
> Hearing loss is just one aspect of who I am. I'm comfortable with myself. I have skills, smarts, and love to share.

If you're looking for an honest person to have fun and maybe a future with, the needs-to-know time starts *as soon as possible*. If not on the first date, then definitely the second date, because by the third date, the new romantic interest will have figured it out already and wonder why you haven't brought it up.

Know your dating deal-breakers. Let's say your new interest suggests a restaurant that you dread because of its darkness and noisiness. You can either suffer through it and not hear well (and we all know how that goes) or suggest in advance that because of your hearing loss, a different spot would be better. If your date insists on going to the first restaurant, wish them a good life and move on.

If you like someone enough to keep dating them, be strong and disclose your hearing loss. Your vulnerability may inspire them to be just as open.

I had an idea that I thought would help with love in the dark, but the Hearing Husband won't wear glow-in-the-dark lipstick.

LIFE TOGETHER: EMBRACE THE HEARING CHALLENGES

What's easier—dealing with hearing loss that started *before* the romantic relationship, or when it occurs or worsens *during* the relationship?

If Shari had known she would not be able to easily hear her husband as her hearing loss progressed, would she have married him? Yes, the many wonderful aspects of their lives together outweigh the challenges. But to make things work, they must continually learn to communicate with each other, over and over again.

This became clear when their daughter was very young. They were enjoying a beautiful day at a lake, when suddenly she was stung by a bee. Being new parents, Shari and her husband did the only logical thing—they completely panicked. Shari would say something. Her husband would mumble a reply. "What did you say?" Shari shouted. He repeated himself but no louder than before. "I can't hear you!" Shari bellowed back.

In a crisis, communication had completely broken down. They needed to do better.

Hearing loss doesn't work on a preferred time schedule. It doesn't hold off its grand entrance until two people have established a relationship that can handle the extra pressure. It happens when it happens, and when it does—*pow*! Life changes and relationships must adapt.

You may have emotional scars from a previous relationship because of poor communication or an inattentive partner. It may take time to build trust and confidence that things can be different this time. Alternatively, your former relationship may have been successful, communication-wise, which puts pressure on your new partner to do just as well.

A common scenario is the couple that has lived together for years. One develops hearing loss only to realize that their partner is a quiet mumbler. The hearing partner is now under pressure to change their way of speaking, and the pair needs to overhaul their interactions—not easily done without frustration, impatience, and a few hurt feelings.

It can be devastating when one partner's hearing loss causes major changes in a relationship:

- You may fear that hearing loss will impact your partner's love for you.

- Your social life as a couple may change.

- There may be grief for the joy of shared activities and the ease of communication you once had.

But hearing loss does not have to be the beginning of the end. Like other relationship-challenging events, you can survive it by taking the time to acknowledge the challenge and working together to adopt whatever is required. In this case, it's a new way of communicating.

What are the ground rules? Many of the suggestions in the section "Recruiting Your Family to Your Team" in Chapter 20 apply here, with the following additions:

Create your own signals. A particularly meaningful look in your partner's direction or a finger alongside your nose can indicate you are having trouble hearing or need a repeat. With practice, your partner will recognize the look of confusion on your face and step in with a repeat before your finger even starts to move. Being attentive to each other's facial expressions and body language will help you communicate better and strengthen your emotional bond.

Set ground rules for group conversations. Decide if and when your partner can let others know about your hearing loss and when and how you want them to repeat what others have said. And then follow the rules. Make new ones as needed.

List your personal communication dos and don'ts. Start with the communication best practices in Chapter 17 and tailor them to your life. You could include rules like:

- No calling out from the other room.

- The person starting the conversation is the one to move closer to the other.

- No talking when the water is running.

Create workarounds that work for you both. Figure out how to make favorite activities enjoyable again. Experiment with technology fixes, use HEAR (hearing check, evaluate, articulate, revise and remind), go to events earlier or later, or whatever works.

Develop ways to cope with the frustration of repeats. Learn how to diffuse anger or how to ask for a break in the action to calm down. Consider seeing a counselor if necessary and follow the rules for arguing with hearing loss discussed later in this chapter.

Involve your partner in your hearing loss life. Take them to your HCP appointments and discuss the barriers you are facing. The more your partner understands about your hearing loss, the more helpful they can be. Introduce them to your hearing loss peers as well. They may learn useful tricks you can try in your own conversations.

Accept that communication will take more work. Hearing loss takes a toll and that's just a fact of your life together. Accept it and make it work.

SEX: KEEPING THE LIGHTS ON CAN BE FUN

People with hearing loss don't *do* dark. When the lights go out, so does the conversation. Disembodied words don't make sense and can cause anxiety, which doesn't spark romance. Hearing people can pillow talk with the lights on or off, and it can be the same for people who are "deafer in the dark," but they may need to be creative. Gael had an idea for a fun way to help with love in the dark, but the Hearing Husband didn't want to wear glow-in-the-dark lipstick.

But who says the lights *have* to be out for pillow talk anyway? Dimmed lights may be romantic, but you can also choose to keep the lights bright, say everything that you want to say, and then turn out the lights for whatever comes next. (Or keep them on—it's your romance!) This calls for some honest couple-conversation so that neither of you miss or misunderstand anything that can lead to, sigh, yet another disagreement.

But if your communication issues spill over into your intimate life, discuss it outside the bedroom first. Then enjoy practicing the perfect combination of romance and communication.

Before he even became the Hearing Husband, Doug clearly didn't see hearing loss in bed as posing any problem—because that's where he proposed! Since Gael removes her hearing devices and corrective lenses when she goes to bed, she wakes up deaf and with blurry vision. But when she opened her eyes one morning, he was only a pillow away and she could see him clearly. He had an odd little smile and then his lips moved in a short but complete sentence. She *saw* him say, "Let's get married."

She didn't want to embarrass herself by answering yes to a question he hadn't asked—her speechreading is great but not perfect—so she asked him if he had just suggested they get married. He mouthed yes, so she did too. Poor guy, if he had known that people with hearing loss around the world would hear about this uniquely timed proposal, he may not have asked!

MAKE IT A FAIR FIGHT

How well do you consider your partner's frustrations? Gael's husband could tell a million stories about the effect of her hearing loss on his life, but he sees it as part of their marriage. However, he still has issues about the time she locked him out of their condo by mistake. She could not hear his desperate attempts—for forty-five minutes—to get back in. Gael thinks it's a funny story. Her husband does not.

Arguments are a fact in most relationships. A positive outcome of a quarrel can clear the air of lingering resentment. However, to be fair for the person with hearing loss, the *format* of your arguments needs to be tweaked. The following guidelines can create a level playing field:

Make sure you can see each other. If you can't see your partner's face, you are at a disadvantage, which might make you angrier. Plus, miscommunications are more likely. Fight facing each other and use good lighting and minimal background noise.

Speak one at a time. Take turns speaking and try not to yell. Overly loud speech is hard to decipher because of the noise and the distortion of the yeller's lips. Smiling is also difficult when you're shouting. But if you must yell, yell one at a time.

Use a normal tone of voice. When a hearing person is asked to repeat themselves, they should use their usual tone of voice—with no over-enunciation or eyeball-rolling—or consider a different choice of words to express the same thought.

Remember, you may be frowning. Be aware that if you usually frown as you speechread, this may be misinterpreted as annoyance, which could make your partner angrier.

In some situations, hearing loss has such a devastating impact on a couple's relationship that outside counseling may be beneficial. Ask your HCP for support or, if they cannot provide it, for a reference to a relationship counselor.

22

PARENTING SAFELY
AND SOUNDLY

ALL PARENTS WORRY about keeping their child safe. A parent with hearing loss has an extra level of worry: *Could my hearing loss cause harm to my child?*

The list of potential dangers is long: not hearing your child crying or when the tone of their voice indicates distress; not being able to locate the voice of a three-year-old who has gotten away from you; unusual sounds like, say, water running when it shouldn't be. Or simply not understanding what your child is trying to say to you.

When hearing loss–related incidents happened with Gael's son, Joel, she cursed herself as a bad mommy who should never have been allowed to bear children. When her toddler got out of her sight for what she could have sworn was only a very short period of time, he managed to turn on the kitchen's hot water tap! Another time, she didn't hear her crawling baby scooch across the rug and out the bedroom door. She ran after him and did a floor dive to catch his feet before her baby ski-jumped down the stairs. As they lay there panting, he laughed and Gael cried.

Deep down, she knew that all mommies, hearing or not, have similar terrifying moments. But, like all parents, she had to learn on the job, as did her son. When Joel was little, he referred to Gael's hearing aids as "hearrings," and he grew up knowing that if he wanted something from mom, he had to communicate in the right way.

When her son was in his early teens, Gael asked him how her hearing loss had affected him. He replied, "Well, always having to repeat myself is kind of irritating. And when you yell at me because of something you thought I said, but you misheard. Oh yeah, and when I'm sitting in the back seat and I almost put my neck out, so you see my lips in the rearview mirror. Stuff like that."

He went on, "But it's okay! If my friends laughed because you misheard me or said something weird, I told them to shut up. Dad and I are proud of you, Mom." That earned him extra rations at dinner that night.

As supportive as your hearing children may be, expect some trick-playing! If you think that your child isn't talking behind your back or jumping around making faces at you—well, they are. Hearing loss can be an object of good-natured fun in the family, like any other condition, but there's a thin line between teasing and tears. Help them to understand the difference.

TIPS FOR PARENTING WITH HEARING LOSS

Parenting, in general, is an ongoing battle for communication— especially once they hit the teen years. No matter their age, sometimes children follow communication best practices and sometimes they don't. They are clear communicators for one sentence but turn away for the next. It can cause sadness and frustration on both sides. You wonder why they can't consistently speak so you can understand them, and they get annoyed that their nagging parent cannot hear them. It is a struggle.

"Remember to face me when you talk to me."

"Please move your hands away from your mouth."

"Come here if you need to talk to me, I can't hear you in another room."

Shari sounds like a broken record, but what is the alternative if she wants to teach her children how to speak so she can understand them? It's not an easy task.

Maybe our expectations are too high. It is difficult for most adults to alter their speech patterns on a regular basis, why should we expect this from children? But on the other hand, childhood is the time when learning is easiest, and new habits are formed daily. They have learned how to hold a fork, dress and bathe on their own, and many other things. Why can't they learn to speak in a loud and clear voice so we can hear them? Some questions have no answers.

How can you remain a patient and loving parent while coping with the added frustration of hearing loss? The first step is to take care of yourself. You'll need the stamina, especially when your children are young.

Here are some other tips:

Teach them about hearing loss. When your children understand what your hearing technology does, the devices become normal and carry no shame. They might even think your technology is cool. Let your children know that if they want you to understand them, they must face you, speak clearly, and use other best practices.

Use visuals. There is no replacement for hyper-vigilance about where your small child is. Audible alerts, such as baby monitors, need to be augmented with visible alerts. Consider a multiroom video alert system to keep tabs on their whereabouts. Or go low-tech with a convex mirror that lets you keep an eye on them in another part of the room. An extra, angled rearview mirror lets you check that back seat passengers are okay.

Be persistent. Parenting is all about repetition. Teach them how to communicate with you; for example, getting your attention before speaking and making sure they are looking at you. Remind them and remind them and, when they forget, remind them again. While it's not always easy, keeping your voice neutral and calm during the reminders is critical.

Encourage them. Notice when they do something to help you hear and compliment them for it; for instance, when they assist in a hard-to-hear encounter at a store or restaurant, or on the phone. Positive reinforcement makes them happy to be your allies.

Forgive them when they fail. We all fail to communicate well from time to time. Staying angry is useless. You can't expect perfection, so use your reminders wisely. This will reduce message fatigue where they just tune you out. And when you do get angry out of frustration, apologize. Older children will begin to empathize with your struggles.

Set boundaries. If something is important to discuss and isn't time sensitive, put it off until you have the necessary energy to communicate at your best. When your children are angry or upset, ask them to calm themselves first and then speak. This not only makes the child easier to understand, but it is an important life skill, too.

Remember to laugh. A joke can lighten a tough situation and prepare everyone to try again. Sometimes mishearings are funny, too. The more comfortable you are with your hearing issues, the more normal they will seem.

Good communication with your children is the goal, not that they follow some specific formula for talking to you. Stay flexible and ask them for ideas about what might work. The good news is that children are accepting. One day Shari asked her children if it bothered them to have a mom with hearing loss. They looked at her like they didn't understand the question. It is all they have ever known.

23

FRIENDS WILL STAY, FRIENDS WILL GO

I N ANY SERIOUS life challenge, you quickly figure out who your real friends are when you need to ask more from them. Just because your friends are nice people doesn't mean they can handle your communication needs. One friend might be soft spoken, and despite your requests to speak up, she finds it difficult and feels like she is yelling. Stepping outside the comfort zone of lifelong behavior is not easy for most people.

The best friends in Gael's life became and remain those who can deal with her constant requests for repeats and need to sit in the middle. Any friend who signs on for the long haul is a person who she can understand and who can understand her. Her friends accept her hearing loss as part of their communication landscape.

After saying something, one friend would immediately repeat it, just to avoid hearing Gael say pardon yet again. It made Gael laugh but also secretly irked her because it reminded her how much she asked people to repeat themselves in those pre-hearing aid days. When she got new hearing aids, she realized that her friends speak more loudly to her than to other people. She's still not quite comfortable asking people to lower their voices—because they're bellowing to help her!

When people are easier to understand—when they speak loudly enough, enunciate their words, and make eye contact—becoming close to them feels easier. Establishing a rapport with people who mumble or cover their mouths when they speak can feel arduous. If the pitch of their voice is difficult to discern, or they fidget or swallow their words or laugh and talk at the same time, you will spend more energy figuring out the words they are saying than the meaning behind them.

Whether hearing loss occurred before or after the start of a friendship may be a factor in how well the friendship thrives. When Shari first started telling her friends about her hearing loss, most of them had no real reaction. They didn't care, which is nice, but they also didn't do much to help her hear. Perhaps they tried for a few minutes and then fell back into their old speaking patterns. That's human nature. Over time, some friends consistently tried, and those are the ones she is closest to today.

Coaching your friends on communication best practices may change some of their behavior, but it may not permanently alter how they speak, especially as they will use their "natural" voice when they talk to other people. When you've been friends with someone for a long time, you have a history that's not going to fall to pieces because of hearing loss. But if a communication partner cannot regularly make the needed changes, sadly, the friendship is likely to wane.

FRIENDS WHO SUPPORT YOU

Friends who understand your hearing needs will reinforce your belief that friendship transcends disability. They help you hear them. They accept the reality of always having to look at you when they talk. They laugh at the mishearings as long as you do, too. And they hold your hand and listen when you share your frustrations and fears.

They may also provide practical assistance such as alerting you to sounds you need to hear or to the fact that someone is speaking to you. Maybe they point discreetly (or not so discreetly) to let you know who. They let you be in charge of how, when, and if you disclose your hearing issues to others, and, when necessary, they will explain it clearly and simply to others.

Hearing loss can help you make friends, too. This can be a temporary friend, like a seatmate on the plane who promises to tell you if the captain says anything important in an emergency, or a considerate waiter who repeats the specials in a way you understand. Other times it can be someone you meet in a Facebook group about hearing loss who provides the perfect suggestion or words of support at the right time. Or even a new acquaintance at a retreat or other special event. Whether in the moment or for the long term, these temporary hearing buddies can be lifesavers.

At a recent yoga retreat, Shari met one such person. At dinner the first night, Shari mentioned to those seated near her that she might have trouble hearing in the crowded space. "Please don't think I am rude if I don't respond appropriately to a question or if I ignore it altogether," she said. "It's only because I didn't hear you. Just tap me and please try again." Everyone was friendly and attentive, and one woman really took this to heart.

At class the next day, Shari's new friend set up her yoga mat right next to hers. Anytime Shari lagged behind, her buddy would turn towards her so Shari could see her lips as she mouthed the instructions. Or she might reach over and move Shari's leg to the right spot. Shari didn't ask her to do any of this, but she found it incredibly helpful. And it made her laugh.

24

TAPPING THE POWER OF PEERS

THERE IS A stunning sense of relief in connecting with another person who has felt the shock of hearing loss. Gael entered her first hearing loss conference as one person and exited as another. It was one big *aha* moment after another. On the final night, a few attendees went to a pub together. The room was empty except for a table of four or five people in the corner. Almost nothing on earth is louder than a dozen people with hearing loss having drinks. Gael was a bit embarrassed by the stares they were drawing from the other, presumably "hearing," bar patrons.

And then it happened. A MindShift! Gael thought, *So what if we are loud? We have hearing loss, yes. And we are also enlightened HoHs enjoying each other's company.* It was a life-changing moment that still resonates for Gael. She went home and looked at her husband with pity. *Poor man. You can hear.*

Heading to her first hearing loss convention, Shari was worried she would not fit in. She didn't yet define herself as someone with hearing loss. If anything, she was still in denial, actively trying to hide her hearing loss much of the time. Finding a peer group changed all that.

Shari's new hearing loss friends showed her there was nothing shameful about hearing loss and taught her tips and tricks she still uses today. They inspired her to advocate for her needs and for the needs of other people with hearing loss, too. Most importantly, she no longer felt alone with her hearing loss. She became part of a community of people like her.

Hearing loss peers can be an incredible source of validation, support, and knowledge. They get it. They are happy to commiserate with you and offer another perspective on hearing loss: one of empowerment and levity. The hearing loss community can be your strongest pillar of support, especially on those bad-hearing days.

Any get-together of hearing loss people, regardless of numbers, takes a little while to get going. It's a not-so-delicate dance designed to make sure everyone is in the best seat for their hearing issues. Some people can't face the window because the light makes it hard to speechread; others prefer people to sit only on their good side. Technology must be compatible and running smoothly for everyone—that's the rule. All this adjusting is done with a smile, or at least an acceptance that this is what *works*. Although it may sound busy, this activity creates a relaxing, stress-free environment for people who struggle to keep up with conversations in the hearing world.

While friendships with some hearing loss peers may begin because of your shared experience with hearing loss, over time your relationships will likely grow as you discover other common interests. Either way, your life will be richer for having met the people who truly understand an important part of who you are.

HOW TO CONNECT WITH HEARING LOSS PEERS

At the start of your hearing loss journey, you may not know other people with hearing loss and may even be reluctant to identify yourself with others based solely on hearing. *I don't need more friends, and I don't join clubs, especially ones with a lot of people moaning about their hearing loss.* That may be stigma talking, or the mistaken belief that an HCP can provide all the necessary information.

Reaching out to hearing loss peers doesn't require a commitment, just the willingness to learn from other people. Some may be ahead of you on the journey's path and can provide the wisdom they have garnered along the way.

Start online by following a hearing loss blog. (Check out Shari's at livingwithhearingloss.com and Gael's at hearinghealthmatters.org/betterhearingconsumer.) Or join a social media group of people with hearing loss. (Shari's group, also called Living With Hearing Loss, is on Facebook.) Many are excellent sources of support and answers. Be aware, though, that some sites share misinformation, including claims of a cure. Be discerning about which are legitimate and do your best to ignore the angry types who just like to vent.

For education and inspiration, nothing beats attending an in-person gathering, whether locally or at a national conference, at least once. You will learn more in a day or a weekend than you can from a year of researching different strategies and options for your hearing loss life online.

Many times in her hearing loss journey, Shari wondered if her life would ever be the same. *Will I be able to achieve my personal and professional goals? Will my relationships suffer?* Meeting other people with hearing loss who led successful, productive, and happy lives was such a relief. She was inspired by their resilience, and it gave her hope that she could accomplish the same.

Hearing loss support groups exist around the world. Your HCP may be able to refer you to a local group, but if not, your best bet is to search for one online. The International Federation of Hard of Hearing People lists member organizations from more than forty countries on its website, IFHOH.org.

Some countries, such as the United States, have several consumer organizations, the largest being Hearing Loss Association of America (HLAA) with more than one hundred local chapters that meet regularly. HLAA also holds an annual convention. Other large organizations include Britain's Hearing Link and RNID, the Canadian Hard of Hearing Association (CHHA), Australia's Soundfair, and the New Zealand Hearing Association, to name a few. The European Federation of Hard of Hearing People (EFHOH) has contact information on European organizations that support people with hearing loss.

Many organizations hold monthly, quarterly, or annual meetings with educational speakers on a variety of hearing loss topics, for example: strategies for living successfully with hearing challenges, managing hearing loss in the workplace, and accessing public and government services. Presentations are often preceded or followed by time for socializing.

Many groups take on local projects like advocating for hearing loops in public spaces, for more affordable technology, and for providing captioning in theaters and cinemas. Some organizations offer confidential peer mentoring programs that connect you with another person with hearing loss who can answer your questions and share their experiences. Even if an organization doesn't offer a formal program, you could ask if a member is willing to work with you one on one.

We encourage you to give a few meetings a try. You have nothing to lose and much to gain from looking into a support organization.

25

IN THE WORKPLACE

THERE ARE SO many employment issues related to hearing loss
that we would need to write a separate book to cover them all!
That book would be a comprehensive guide to navigating communication access in all the work-related processes of applying for
jobs, being hired, training, and then doing your job. Employees
with disabilities have rights, but they often have to fight for them.

This book is *not* that book. Instead, in this chapter, the focus
is on disclosure and establishing a support team among your
coworkers. The next part of this book, Hearing Hacks, offers tips
for effective communication on the job, including how to handle
meetings, placement of office furniture, and so on.

DISCLOSING YOUR HEARING LOSS AT WORK

For most of Shari's career in finance, she hid her hearing loss
from almost everyone, including her boss. In the early days, when
her hearing loss was mild enough, she could secretly pop in her
hearing aids right before important meetings and take them out

immediately after. She lived in fear that her batteries would die, leaving her incapacitated in front of her colleagues. Her secret weighed on her, and she began avoiding hard-to-understand colleagues and clients (not the best career move), until one fateful meeting with an important new client.

The new CEO of a large retail company was clearly under the weather, with watery eyes, a cough, and a weaker than normal voice. "I'll sit across the table from you," he said, "so I don't pass on this cold." This was a thoughtful gesture, but as Shari sized up the vast expanse of conference table now between them, she worried she wouldn't be able to hear him. As he began to answer her first question, her fears were realized—she couldn't understand a word he said.

She hadn't yet begun disclosing her hearing loss to people, preferring to fake it when she couldn't hear. But that strategy was not going to cut it here. Having no choice, she took a deep breath and came clean. "I don't hear well, so it would be better if we sat closer to one another," she said. "I will have to take my chances with your cold." Laughing, he moved closer, and the meeting was a success, especially because she didn't get sick. The positive experience made Shari wish she had been braver about revealing her hearing loss in other situations, too.

Managing the challenges of hearing loss in the workplace starts with disclosure. Stigma may be holding you back and even when you *do* decide to disclose, you may find that your employer is not familiar with the technology and practices needed for the communication aspects of your job. But if your employer doesn't know about your communication challenges, you may appear to struggle in some work situations but thrive in others, confusing your colleagues and clients, who may have limited knowledge of hearing loss. Disclosing is an important first step towards better work performance as well as job satisfaction.

> ### MindShift
> **Being open about my hearing loss will help me communicate better. Trying to hide my hearing loss leads to misunderstandings.**

It's When, Not If

Your decision to disclose your hearing loss to employers, current or prospective, is a "when" and not an "if." Our advice about when to disclose is . . . it depends. Being honest about who you are, your strengths and weaknesses, is always a good personal policy. But in certain life areas, such as employment, the timing is critical.

Neither a resume nor a job application is the place to disclose your hearing loss; the purpose in either is strictly for you to show why you are best suited for the job. Unfortunately, declaring a disability may cause some prospective employers to put your application into the "thanks, but no thanks" pile. Although this is illegal, it does happen—and can be very difficult to prove.

Many workplace professionals recommend the first interview as the best place and time to disclose your hearing loss; you got the interview based on your background and skills, and this is the opportunity to cement their opinion of you in person. Rather than hiding your hearing loss—and risking the interviewers suspecting it, even though they are not allowed to ask you about it—you have a golden opportunity to demonstrate that, with effective support, your hearing loss was not a hindrance in previous jobs and can even contribute to *better* communication in the workplace. Highlight your skills rather than your disability. Of course, if you need accommodation for the interview, request it in advance.

In first interviews, Gael could not get through a conversation, which often involved two or more interviewers, without disclosing. So, after the initial chit-chat, she would say, "I have hearing loss, and I use hearing technology. Also, I need to see your faces while we're talking." She said this confidently (even if she was nervous) and with a smile, putting them at ease with her hearing loss. At some point during the interview, she would say something like, "In my previous work, my hearing loss didn't interfere with my being able to do a good job."

You may choose to wait until your second interview or after you get the job. But if you bluff your way through your first interview, you risk misunderstanding the questions, answering inappropriately, and not properly hearing the answers to *your* questions so that you can make an informed decision about whether this is the right workplace for you.

Regardless of the stage you choose to self-identify, let your employer know what you need to enhance communication in your position, which, it's important to remember, you were hired for on merit. If you don't know what will help you, find out. (See the "Hearing Hacks" section of the book for suggestions.) The costs and inconvenience for you to do your job well are often minimal, and it is your employer's job to support you.

If your hearing loss begins when you are already on the job, perhaps in a place where you've been working for some time, the same honesty-is-the-best policy applies. Chances are your coworkers may already suspect you have hearing loss. Or they may think something else is wrong—that you have emotional issues, that you're not smart, or that you're a poor listener. What they know for sure is that something is amiss.

When Shari was first promoted into a management role, she was excited about her new responsibilities. But she didn't realize that a big part of a manager's job is listening to other people's secrets. Trouble with your colleagues? Talk to management. Disappointed with your year-end bonus? Talk to management. Need time off to care for your ailing parent? Talk to management. All day long, people shared confidential information with her in hushed tones. *Can I ask people to repeat their secrets—only louder this time?* she wondered. Luckily her office was quiet, and she could ask clarifying questions, but being open about her hearing issues would have made her job much easier.

The good news is that strong work performance usually speaks for itself. Disclosing your hearing issues will not change your hard-won reputation, especially if you have been on the job for some time. And it will ease the pressure of having to hear everything perfectly. Being open about your hearing loss will help your colleagues understand why you may require certain accommodations, such as changing an office layout or introducing new technology. When you can explain in clear and unemotional language the communication basics that you need to stay connected, everyone benefits.

Plus, authenticity is often rewarded. Your honesty gives your colleagues permission to open up about their own challenges, too, helping you to forge stronger relationships. And there it is—your support network!

FINDING WORKPLACE SUPPORT

You must understand your needs before asking for support. When Gael moved to a new city, she made her *least* self-aware career move ever; she took a job as a receptionist for a professional accounting association. She had no problem with the acting professional part, but it was the how-to-hear-clearly-on-the-phone part that didn't work out well. It was an era of almost no available assistive technology, but she had told her employer that, in spite of her hearing loss, she could handle the switchboard. When it was apparent that she could *not* hear well enough for the demands of the job, she and her employer agreed to call it quits. She ran out the door with relief, resolving never again to take a job that wasn't suited to her.

The changing times are good for people with hearing loss. Millennials and subsequent generations are more knowledgeable, and often more understanding, about disabilities and the people who have them. In school, it has become more common to give students with learning differences extra time on tests and other accommodations. This exposure and emerging openness bode well for increased accessibility in the workplace.

The law is also often on your side. Some countries have legislation that mandates employers to provide "reasonable accommodations" for employees with hearing loss, as long as it does not cause "undue hardship" for the employer, which is defined as significant difficulty or expense. Reasonable accommodations could include things like captioned phones, assistive listening devices, or work area adjustments like a change in seating location.

Some workplaces also have employee-led disability forums or other groups that provide mentorship, assistance in finding solutions for you to perform your job well, and camaraderie with others facing similar challenges. Many employers are committed to creating diverse and inclusive workplaces, and you can educate leaders with your personal expertise on how to be inclusive of people with hearing loss.

Remember, you are your own best advocate. Don't make your hearing loss solely your employer's "problem"; it's a shared issue. Understanding your needs and knowing your rights as an employee with a disability will help you disclose and obtain the access you need. Research the tools and workarounds that support you doing your job and ask for those specific items. Your job performance and enjoyment depend on it.

26

CHOOSING THE RIGHT HCP

WHEN SHARI FIRST began having trouble hearing, she was not an expert on communication best practices. She thought that her audiologist would share a broad range of information with her, including things like accessibility options for watching TV or attending movies or the theater. But her first HCP focused the conversation solely on devices. What type of hearing aid did she want, and what was her budget?

An audiologist with a different approach could have eased Shari's transition to living with hearing loss and saved a lot of frustration and sadness. Today, Shari seeks out HCPs who extend their focus beyond the technical aspects of audiograms and hearing aid fittings to the emotional aspects of hearing loss—ones who take the time to understand Shari's specific communication needs and plan her treatment to include new technologies.

Gael's current audiologists have more influence on her peace of mind and quality of life than anyone who is not a husband, child, or important friend. She sees her hearing professional more frequently than she sees her family doctor, because her hearing loss requires more attention and poses more barriers than any other health challenge. Her audiologist is a trusted advisor on her key technical supports, her hearing aid, and her cochlear implant.

But, like Shari, that wasn't always the case. One long-ago HCP stopped Gael mid-hearing test and said, "I don't think you're trying hard enough." Others were dismissive of strategies outside the realm of the hearing aid. On the rare occasion when, in talking about her hearing loss, Gael cried, the practitioners waited for her to calm herself and then went on without addressing the raw emotion that was happening right there, in their office—a missed opportunity to provide much-needed support and advice. In another memorable appointment, Gael started to cry as she talked about her new and devastating tinnitus, and the recently graduated audiologist started to cry, too. Gael ended up soothing *her.*

Now Gael has a hand-picked team of professionals who provide solid, helpful services. They also remind her that she may not know as much as she thinks she does about hearing loss—*they* are still the experts on many aspects. And she reminds *them* to respect the wisdom of the real-life experience she brings to the professional-client relationship.

The ideal HCP practices person-centered care. This means they work to understand your individual communication challenges and partner with you to solve them. They ask important questions and listen to your answers. They show empathy for your struggles. Your input, along with their expertise, is crucial in finding solutions that work best for you.

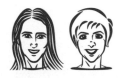

The best HCPs are communication specialists who create personalized solutions that include both technology and non-technical strategies.

A successful relationship must be based on mutual trust and a united focus on creating better communication outcomes. This requires establishing a working relationship with clearly defined goals and a plan of action. This is a win for everyone—you *and* your HCP.

THE BEST HCP FOR YOU

The best HCPs are true communication specialists, creating solutions that include hearing aids as well as assistive listening devices and even direct-to-consumer devices or apps like the ones discussed in the "Technology" section of this book.

When you first meet, your HCP must learn who you are before they can help you. You are a unique individual with hearing difficulties and priorities and are likely using a homegrown mix of communication skills and technical knowledge. Your personality, emotional background, and life situations dictate your response to hearing loss.

Whether you are new to hearing loss or have been using hearing aids for years, you have choices and input into decisions involving your *aural rehabilitation*: a fancy term for learning how to communicate and live better with hearing loss. At every meeting with your HCP, there should be a two-way conversation, an exchange of information. At appropriate times, you'll discuss different communication strategies, including assistive technology. At no point should you be *told* what to do or when to do it, nor that this-hearing-aid-here is the best and only option for you.

You and your HCP need to be a good fit. Consider the following factors in your search:

Personality. Because you will work closely with this professional, you must feel comfortable with them. They should be honest, set realistic expectations, and speak plainly without overusing jargon so you can understand. Be certain, though, to differentiate between resistance to your hearing loss and resistance to the HCP.

Good communication skills. If there's one person you should be able to understand, it's your hearing care professional! Surprisingly, some HCPs don't use best practice communication skills like speaking with sufficient volume while facing you, which can cause extra stress. Alert your HCP if you are not understanding them well, and if the problem persists consider working with someone else.

Listening ability. The best communication skill an HCP can possess is the ability to actively listen to you, to not only hear what you articulate but to pick up on what you convey through emotion and actions. To listen well, the professional needs to know which questions will elicit information they need to best treat you.

Location and hours of operation. Where possible, choose an HCP with a convenient office location and flexible operating hours. Once you are settled in with your hearing devices, you may not be visiting as often, but if a problem arises, you will want quick access.

Robust product offerings. An HCP should not promote just one brand of hearing aid. Most hearing aid brands offer excellent products, each with unique sound quality and programming features; therefore, one brand will not work for every client. Choose an HCP who offers a variety of options so you can work together to find the most suitable product.

Ethical business practices. Reputable HCPs will let you try a new pair of hearing aids or other devices for at least thirty days. Sixty days is even better. (In many jurisdictions, a sufficient trial period is standard practice required by the industry's governing body.) They will not press you to buy something you cannot afford and may even offer financing solutions. If your professional doesn't meet these basic conditions, find someone else.

Qualifications. Expect training and professionalism. Only commit to the care of an HCP who has the appropriate credentials for your country. Audiologists typically hold a master's degree or doctorate, while hearing instrument specialists should be graduates of a two-to-three-year focused training program.

HOW TO SUPPORT THIS PARTNERSHIP

Hearing health professionals cannot perform miracles. You must actively participate in the process. Be cooperative, open-minded, and honest with your HCP. The more you contribute—and the more questions you ask—the better the outcomes will be. Here's how you can support this important partnership:

Share your hearing loss story and struggles. This is not the time to play tough guy. The more you reveal about your personal challenges, the more information your HCP will have when planning possible solutions.

Come armed with facts. Keep detailed notes about how you are hearing in a variety of situations with your hearing aids so you can assist your HCP with any necessary fine-tuning. The more specific data you can provide—the location, time of day, communication partner, decibel level, and so on—the better.

Leave anger at home. Hearing loss is frustrating, and although hearing aids help a lot, they are not perfect solutions. Try to maintain an analytical attitude towards your communication issues. Anger won't solve problems and may prevent you from finding a creative solution.

Properly maintain hearing devices. Keeping your aids in top condition will prolong their lifespan and help you hear your best.

Respect your HCP's expertise. Although you know the most about your experiences and communication desires, HCPs use time-tested diagnostic tools and programming methods. Blending the two areas of expertise is the best way to find a dynamic solution.

Honor the journey. Your relationship with your hearing loss and your HCP may change over time as you accept your hearing difficulties and learn the types of assistance that you need. Be open to sharing new insights and attitudes along the way.

Teach what you know. When you discover new tricks or useful apps that make hearing easier for you in a certain situation, share them with your HCP, who can then spread the word to other clients. Similarly, you can benefit from the experience of other clients.

Stay in touch. Regular hearing aid checkups are a good time to inquire about new assistive technology—and to let your HCP know of any changes to your hearing situation. Regular visits allow you to keep tabs on your hearing loss, keep your devices fresh, and stay current on new developments.

HEARING HACKS
Putting It All Together

GAEL: So far, we have focused on the theory of communicating better—understanding the big picture, shifting your mental approach, the magic of technology, managing relationships, and various powerful nontechnical tools like HEAR.

 SHARI: Now it's time for the nitty-gritty. Let's put these ideas to work. We call these Hearing Hacks—

 GAEL: Can I jump in for a moment? We need to clarify what we mean by *hack*. I'm a few years older than Shari, and when we first talked about hacks, I went *whoa!* To me, a hack always meant someone who's not good at their job; for example, if someone didn't like my writing or Shari's, they could call us hack writers. (Obviously they can't, because clearly we're not!) Or you could hack into something, like a computer. But when we say hack here, we mean it in the positive sense of the word. Tell them, Shari...

 SHARI: Hacks are tricks, techniques, or workarounds that make everyday tasks easier. They help us better manage our time or do something more efficiently. There are hacks for peeling an orange (use one long continuous cut around the outside from top to bottom) or chilling white wine in the glass without watering it down (add frozen grapes).

GAEL: And now there are Hearing Hacks! Honestly, there have always been Hearing Hacks, but if nobody told you about them, or if you didn't happen to stumble onto their simple, logical steps on your own, how would you know?

 SHARI: Hearing Hacks make living with hearing loss easier. They are the secret sauce that we share with each other over a glass of wine in a quiet cafe or on captioned Zoom calls. You may already use some of these, or you may use ones that we haven't mentioned.

 GAEL: And this, friends, is the art of living skillfully with hearing loss.

27

HACKS FOR
EVERY OCCASION

BEFORE GETTING INTO specific life activities, there are a few Hearing Hacks that are *so good*, *so important*, and *so simple* that you can apply them to almost everything you do. Some will look familiar—we have discussed them in other parts of the book— but they are *so critical* to success that a little repetition can't hurt:

Self-identify. Always, always, always self-identify! Then, remind, remind, remind! Making others aware of your hearing loss and communication needs is the number one Hearing Hack.

Be prepared. Nobody knows better than you about what can go wrong. Think ahead about where you are going and what you are doing, then prepare to meet the challenges.

Arrive early for everything. You need this time to get your technology organized, get the best seat, and advise whoever needs to know about your hearing loss needs.

Stay battery-stocked and charged. Carry a supply so that you never, ever get caught without a replacement on hand if a battery dies. Technology depends on batteries or electricity to work!

Use assistive listening devices. You have assistive listening devices for a reason. Be willing to experiment with new technologies for better results.

Get a hearing buddy. Using another human for a Hearing Hack is not only allowed but encouraged! Whatever the situation, your hearing buddy can fill in the blanks, alert you to danger, punch you when you're bluffing, or whatever else you need this person to do. This isn't you being *dependent*, it's you being *skillful*.

Choose the best seat. Choose a spot that gives you the best view of the people who will be speaking and any audiovisual content. At meetings with rows of chairs or at places of worship, this often means sitting at the *front*—unless, of course, you are using your T-coil, in which case you can sit anywhere you want, although we still recommend finding a seat with good sightlines.

Use visual signals. Any information that you cannot hear needs to be *seen*. In many activities and social situations, agreed-upon signals can clarify spoken information. Just make sure that you and the other person both understand what the signals mean.

Provide praise and feedback. Wherever and whenever you have asked for accommodations—restaurants, hospitals, tours—let the provider know how it went, offering both praise and suggestions about how they can improve. This is the only way that society will learn how to serve and accommodate people with hearing loss.

Keep your sense of humor. Hearing Hacks delivered with a bit of fun tell the world you are comfortable with your hearing loss and can even see the humor in it. Decorate your hearing aids and sound processors with stick-on bling or wear a T-shirt or a button that says, for example, *Face Me. I Read Lips.* If this is too "out there" for you, just settle for a sense of humor.

And don't forget the mother of all Hearing Hacks. HEAR (hearing check, evaluate, articulate, revise and remind) lets you take charge of any communication situation.

28

SOCIAL EVENTS

Socializing with hearing loss can be a loud and stressful experience. Today's popular restaurant decor includes hardwoods, mirrors, and metal—all surfaces that reflect noise rather than absorb it. At cocktail parties, many voices talking at once will make it hard to pinpoint the voice you are trying to hear. People with hearing loss often opt for an easy out—dominating the conversation or nodding, smiling, and hoping our responses are appropriate.

But that's not you, is it? Use these Hearing Hacks for a more satisfying experience for everyone.

DINING OUT

Choose a quiet place:
- Read restaurant reviews for noise ratings or consult a crowd-sourcing app that ranks restaurants in a geographical area by ease of conversation.

- Use online pictures as clues about the decor's potential for noise. Look for sound-absorbing surfaces like carpets, drapes, cushioned seats, cloth tablecloths, and acoustic tiles.

- Ask others for ideas—everyone is looking for a quieter place these days.

Plan ahead:

- When you make the reservation, specify your needs. Don't just ask for a quiet table. Mention your hearing loss and ask for a table in the corner or by a wall.

- Consider eating at off hours when restaurants are quieter (although dinner at 2 p.m. might be a bit early for some people). Management may be more open to requests like turning down the music at those times.

- Dine outside if the weather permits. Outdoor spaces have fewer hard surfaces to reflect sound and more organic material to absorb it.

- Limit your group's size to four to six people for easier conversation and lipreading.

- Request a round table. Group conversation is easier because everyone will be equally visible for speechreading. Or choose a booth that absorbs sound and contains the conversation to the confined space.

Make environmental changes as needed:

- Become confident in asking for another table (if the first one is inadequate) or for the manager to lower the music.

- Ask to see the specials in writing rather than spoken by the waiter. Alternatively, ask the server to stand close to you and articulate the specials clearly.

Pick the right seat:

- When dining with a large group, seat yourself in the spot that works best for *you*.

- Position yourself in the center to be closer to a larger number of diners.

- Sit with your back to the wall to reduce distracting noise behind you.

- Situate difficult-to-hear people across from you for easier speechreading.

Use technology fixes:

- Ask your HCP to create a restaurant program for your devices that blocks out background noise and focuses on voices.

- Use an assistive listening device that brings voices into your ears, such as a remote microphone that your dinner companions can clip to their clothing or that can be put on the table.

- Use a speech-to-text app to understand what others are saying.

Pay it forward:

- Leave reviews to help other diners find quiet spots and avoid loud ones.

- Reward a good experience with repeat business and recommend the restaurant to friends and family.

SURVIVING LOUD PARTIES AND EVENTS

Take control by volunteering to host:

- Hosting gives you more control over the environment.

- Turn the music down and the lights up.

- Set aside an area for quiet conversations.

- Plan the seating so you have an advantageous spot for communication.

If you are not hosting, arrive early to scope out the scene:

- Ask the host to implement some of the suggestions above in at least one section of the space, including lowering the music to aid with conversation.

- Identify quieter areas conducive to conversation. The best spots are often in a corner where background noise behind you is limited. Look for carpet, drapes, or cushions that can absorb excess sound. Or go outside.

Make the most of a difficult situation:

- Arrive rested and armed with better powers of concentration.

- Take a deep breath, recite a MindShift, and get in there. You deserve to hear and be heard.

- Ask conversation partners to move to a quieter part of the room (see above). Or invite them to step outside for some air and respite from the cacophony.

- Take listening breaks to rest your brain because listening fatigue is real. Help in the kitchen, walk around the block, or retreat to the restroom. Whatever works.

- Use visual cues to indicate you are having trouble hearing. A cupped hand behind your ear will let the speaker know to raise their voice without disrupting the flow of the conversation.

- Show off your tech tools. Speech-to-text apps are interesting to almost everyone.

At a seated dinner, converse strategically:

- You may need to focus on speaking with the people nearest you at the table. Longer-distance conversations may be frustrating and cause more cross-talking and noise.

- Experiment with different programs on your hearing aids or whip out your tech tools. Your conversation partners might enjoy experimenting with new and cutting-edge technologies.

Laugh and enjoy:

- Accept mishears as part of the hearing loss life. Inevitably, you will hear something incorrectly or reply to a question you thought you heard rather than the actual question.

- When you laugh, others will laugh with you. After all, some of those mishears are *really* funny!

29

ENTERTAINMENT

GOING TO THE movies can be daunting for people with hearing loss. Why not wait until the film is streaming online so you can watch it from home with the captions on? Live theater is another challenge. The dialogue moves quickly and the distance from the stage makes it hard to speechread. Plus, the tickets are not cheap! Why spend the money for a performance you might only partially hear?

But don't miss out on the energy of a group event. These Hearing Hacks will help you enjoy the show.

GOING TO THE MOVIES

Select theaters with accessibility options:

- Check local listings for *open captioned performances* where the captions appear directly on the movie screen. These are wonderful but rare.

- Try foreign-language films with subtitles.

- Most movie theaters in the United States and Canada provide free caption reader devices for individual use. Clip one into your cup holder, position the gooseneck so the captions are in your sightline, and enjoy personal captions. Some theaters offer captioned glasses instead.

Test equipment before use:

- Arrive early to pick up your device and troubleshoot any technical issues, such as being connected to the right theater in a multi-cinema complex.

- Before accepting the device, ask the host to confirm the battery level to avoid a mid-movie disappointment.

Bring noise-cancelling headphones:

- This approach won't work for everyone, but if you are sensitive to loud sounds, noise-cancelling headphones can be a lifesaver during a loud film.

- Use a caption reader to fill in the dialogue.

Pay it forward:

- If things went well, let the venue know. Positive feedback highlights how important it is to keep the devices working well.

- When something goes awry, let them know that, too. Be polite and factual, and also explain that you are disappointed that your needs were not met. The only way theater personnel will understand the importance of these devices is if we demonstrate it.

- If there are consistent problems at a particular cinema, report the problem to the corporate office. Changes in training and procedures may be required.

ATTENDING LIVE THEATER

Understand your options:

- Most theaters provide one or more free options for auditory assistance. Opera performances may also have *supertitles*, which are translated captions of lyrics and dialogue that appear above the stage. Availability will vary by location and venue.

- Arrive early to pick up your device of choice. Lines are often long, and devices sometimes run out. Be prepared to leave photo identification as collateral.

- If you have problems with a theater device, alert an attendant during intermission if you're not able to leave your seat without disrupting others.

- Try out different options. Infrared systems, FM systems, hearing loops, and captions are all available. Get to know them and choose what works best for you.

Infrared headsets are the most common:

- Know the drawbacks. With some models, you must remove your hearing aids, which may make the sound level too quiet for your hearing loss. Other models allow the use of neck loops that work with hearing aids.

- Position yourself well; devices work best with a clear sightline to the stage.

FM systems are also often available:

- You wear this type of device around your neck rather than over your ears.

- Connect by plugging in headphones (your own or the theater's) or linking to your hearing aid via the T-coil setting.

- If you prefer to use your own headphones, call to verify the type of headphone connection the system requires.

- Know that headphone volume levels may not be loud enough for people with certain hearing losses.

When they are available, hearing loops offer top-notch sound:

- Set your device to T-coil mode so the sound comes directly into your hearing aid or cochlear implant.

- If your personal devices do not have telecoil, explore hearing loop receiver earphones, which can be used to tap into a hearing loop. You may need to remove your hearing aids to use them.

Open captioned performances, where offered, are usually limited to specific performances:

- Reserve seats with a good sightline to the captions which generally appear on a display board located to one side of the stage.

On-demand captioning devices:

- GalaPro is a smartphone app that provides theater captioning—most notably on Broadway and in London's theater district—after the first four weeks of a show's run.

- Captions appear on your phone rather than on a screen next to the stage. Preprogrammed based on lighting cues, synchronicity with the dialogue is not always perfect.

- Check with your local theater for availability.

- Fully charge your devices in advance if you plan to use them.

- To avoid complaints or misunderstandings, you may want to alert people seated beside and behind you that you will be using your phone for captioning access during the show.

WATCHING TELEVISION

Use closed captions:
- This is the top Hearing Hack for watching TV with hearing loss!

- Captions are accurate and timely on most scripted programs; problems can arise with live programs like the news or sports, where captioning is done in real time by remote captioners.

- If you observe repeated errors on a particular program, report it to the relevant telecommunications agency in your area so improvements can be made.

- Play with display options. If the captions cover the screen or the score of the big game, check the TV's settings because they may allow you to change the display.

- Set family ground rules to avoid arguments. Although captions can be turned on and off, we suggest a basic rule: captions are always on.

Upgrade your sound system:

- Use a sound bar or additional external speaker. Today's thinner TVs often mean shrunken speakers—so small as to seriously compromise sound quality.

- For the best possible sound, use a soundbar containing a third speaker—specifically for dialogue, with independent volume control.

- Sound bars can be expensive and complicated to install, but when you find the right one it's a good investment.

Stream directly from your hearing device via Bluetooth or T-coil:

- Use a TV streaming device to connect Bluetooth-enabled hearing aids or cochlear implants directly to the TV, bringing the sound into your devices, or use Bluetooth-enabled headphones. The downside of this is that real-time talking with your fellow viewers can be difficult as ambient noise is diminished.

- Install a small induction hearing loop in your TV room. Connect to the TV through a telecoil-enabled hearing device or a telecoil-enabled headset.

- New options may soon be available as streaming connectivity is an area of rapid growth in hearing technology.

Use stand-alone (non-streaming) amplification devices:

- TV amplifier systems use a transmitting base that plugs into your television. Connect by wearing a headset (some models may not be suitable for hearing aid users). Adjusting the volume in the headset will not impact the TV volume for others.

- Use a portable speaker to bring the sound closer to you. Plug the transmitter into the TV and place the speaker closer to where you are sitting. Others in the room will hear the sound from these speakers, too, so this may be a better option for solo viewing.

VISITING A MUSEUM OR GALLERY OR TAKING A GUIDED TOUR

Prepare ahead of time to get the right access:
- Consult the venue's website to learn what hearing accommodations are available. Many venues have hearing aid–compatible audio guides.

- Identify a point person on staff who can act as an accessibility coordinator if needed.

- Provide notice if you require something outside the normal scope, and follow up to ensure things are ready for your visit.

Make specific requests:
- You may be the first person to ask for CART (Communication Access Realtime Translation), or for the tour guide to wear a remote microphone.

- Educate and explain with patience. Your self-advocacy benefits everyone!

- If you don't use sign language, let them know, as this is often the default accommodation provided.

- Arrive early to test the equipment.

Refine your process:

- Provide feedback and ask for it as well. What could *you* have done to make it easier for the venue to meet your needs? Incorporate the feedback into your Hearing Hack for next time.

ATTENDING A CONCERT

Protect your residual hearing:

- Concerts can be very loud—a hundred decibels or higher. Even very short periods of exposure can cause permanent hearing damage.

- Wear earplugs to protect your hearing. You want to preserve the hearing you have, and the plugs will not protect your ears if they stay in your bag.

- Wear hearing protection from the concert's start to its finish to stay safe. If you take earplugs out for even a few minutes, you are incurring damage.

- If you go to concerts frequently, consider investing in a pair of custom earplugs that provide better protection.

- Consider musician earplugs, which lower the volume but leave the frequency balance unchanged to maintain sound quality. If removing hearing devices is not an option, change volume levels or other settings on your devices to minimize noise input.

Use earplugs properly:

- Practice inserting earplugs before you go, and explore online guides for proper instructions on using standard foam earplugs. Earplugs won't do their job unless inserted properly.

- Consider using over-the-ear muffs that are designed as hearing protection and which might be more comfortable for you.

Bring extras!

- Offer earplugs to family, friends, and those seated near you. Earplugs are not usually sold at concerts, so the people around you might be grateful for the protection.

30

HEALTH CARE

MEDICAL APPOINTMENTS AND hospital visits are stressful under normal conditions, and even more so for people with hearing loss. When we are nervous, our hearing plunges—or our concentration might fail. What if we miss important details about our care? Provide the wrong answer to an important medical question? What if we don't even realize we didn't hear something properly?

This can powerfully affect your health and well-being. These Hearing Hacks will reduce the risks and smooth the process for you, for your family, and for the medical professionals you see.

MEDICAL APPOINTMENTS

Self-identify:

- Request the accommodations you need when booking the appointment. Ask health care providers to note your hearing loss in your chart for future reference.

- If possible, bring a relative or friend with you. Two pairs of ears are better than one. They can also take notes.

- If you are on your own, ask to be notified personally when it is your turn so you can relax in the waiting area.

- If your doctor is unwilling or unable to communicate effectively, find another one.

Document your needs in writing:

- Complete a communication access plan (CAP) and share it with your providers. A CAP lists the types of devices you use to hear and what you need from health care providers for better communication.

- Ask that your CAP be kept in your medical record for easy access at each appointment, but bring it with you anyway, in case it is misplaced.

- Find a sample CAP on Hearing Loss Association of America's website.[13]

Apply HEAR (hearing check, evaluate, articulate, revise and remind):

- Wear your devices and use assistive listening tools to fill in gaps. Speech-to-text apps work well in medical settings, but paper and pen work, too. Writing notes is basic but effective.

- Remind medical staff to use communication best practices like facing you when speaking. If personal protective equipment is required in the medical setting, request that clear masks be worn to help with speechreading.

- Don't accept poor communication—your health is at stake. Repeatedly advocate for your needs if necessary.

Ask for important details in writing:

- Ask that they note the key conclusions of your visit, including any required medication and dosage information.

- Request all insurance and billing information in writing and ask for clarification when needed.

- Request that they confirm your next appointment via email or text rather than a call.

Request a telehealth appointment:

- If your doctor offers such appointments, they allow you to see the speaker and control the volume of speech.

- Ask if your doctor's virtual platform supports captions (either CART or automatic). If so, request that they turn them on in advance. If not, use your speech-to-text app.

- Remind your doctor or other health professional that you have hearing loss and ask them to speak clearly and maintain eye contact.

HOSPITAL VISITS

Communicate your needs before you go to the hospital:

- If you need accommodations like CART, request this well in advance.

- Be as specific as possible. Hospitals are notorious for assuming sign language interpreters help all patients with hearing loss.

- Provide feedback on the good and the bad so hospitals continue to improve their standards of care.

Use a hearing loss hospital kit. Packaged kits may be available from your local hearing loss association. Or you can build your own kit using the following ideas:

- Include stickers and signs indicating your hearing loss, to be used on your chart and around your hospital bed.

- Pack sheets or cards listing hearing loss communication tips to share with medical staff.

- Bring a brightly colored storage container for your hearing devices so they are not misplaced or discarded when not in use. Label the container with your full name and the number of devices.

- For extra credit: Include a plastic bag labeled with your name and HEARING AIDS printed on it in large letters, and a safety pin. Keep your devices in the bag and pin it to your hospital gown if you need to remove your devices for a procedure outside your room.

Pack your technology go-bag:

- Include any spare hearing aids you have, extra batteries, all chargers, and any additional communication devices that you find helpful.

- Consider leaving your new hearing aids at home if you have a back-up pair that works well enough.

- Electrical outlets may be far from your hospital bed so include an extension cord.

Label your room:

- Hearing loss is invisible and easily forgotten by medical professionals. Hang up signs over your bed and on the door alerting your caregivers about your hearing loss.

- Remind, remind, and remind again. Staff shifts change often, and new people may not be familiar with your communication needs.

Bring a hearing buddy if possible:

- Hospital stays are stressful, and hearing loss brings additional challenges. A friend or family member can be another set of eyes (and ears) to facilitate communication.

- They might notice that you didn't hear something correctly, despite what you thought you heard. Let them support you.

31

ON THE JOB

OMMUNICATION ON THE job is a big area of concern for people with hearing loss. There are many valuable resources available online that cover the application process, working out an accessibility plan with your employer, and other hearing-related topics. Your local or national hearing loss consumer associations are a good resource, as is your HCP.

If you work in an office environment, the following Hearing Hacks will make it easier for you to do your job well. These hacks may also be effective in different work environments, such as retail, warehouse, and health and education service industries.

If these hacks don't seem applicable or adaptable to your job, they might inspire you to create ones specifically for your workplace. Consider using the HEAR (hearing check, evaluate, articulate, revise and remind) strategies and others discussed in this book.

Regardless of your workplace environment, as we discussed, disclosing your hearing loss on the job is an important step.

OFFICE HACKS

Set up your office for success:

- Situate your desk in an area that is quiet and where you can see people approaching. Today's open plan offices create significant background noise.

- Request the office technology you need to do your job well. Adjustable volume headsets are inexpensive and effective. Captioned phones may also be available. Alternatively, use a video conferencing call platform with ASR (automatic speech recognition) captions.

- Add soft surfaces like carpet to your office, if possible. Sound-absorbing materials are preferable, but not always practical in today's hard-surface offices.

Set communication ground rules:

- Do your best to replace audible messages with visual ones. Let colleagues know you prefer email or text over voicemail. Explain this on your outgoing voicemail message as well.

- Remind colleagues to get your attention before speaking to you.

- Share the best practices for communication partners found in Chapter 17.

ATTENDING AN IN-PERSON MEETING

Prepare ahead of the meeting:

- Get the agenda and the primary speaker's notes in advance, if possible, so you know the topics to be covered and any new words or phrases that will be discussed.

- Ask the organizer if a microphone can be used at the meeting. This benefits everyone and will minimize interruptions and cross-talk if people need to use the mic to speak.

- If you plan to request accommodations like CART, do so at least a week in advance. Formal accommodations may be hard to arrange for impromptu sessions.

Choose the best seat:

- As you would do when dining out (see tips in Chapter 28), arrive early so you can choose the best seat. Sitting at the center position of a table will place you closer to other participants.

- Avoid positioning yourself near sources of extraneous noise like the air conditioner or electronic equipment that hums.

- If you can organize the seating, place the people hardest for you to hear directly across from you so you can see their faces for lipreading.

Use assistive listening technology:

- Remote mics bring distant voices directly into your devices.

- Speech-to-text apps also work well for filling in words you miss. Check before using a speech-to-text app to make sure it is in line with company policy. Some that create permanent transcripts may not be allowed.

Follow up to make sure you got it right:

- Borrow other attendees' written notes to fill in any information you missed.

- If slides were used, request a copy of them, along with presentation notes if possible.

- Send or ask for an email summary of the meeting, including to-dos and other follow-up items. Everyone will appreciate this opportunity to clarify and confirm next steps.

PHONE AND VIDEO CONFERENCE CALLS

Follow the in-person meeting rules above related to preparation and follow-up.

Request video calls rather than audio-only calls whenever possible:

- Video conference calls provide valuable lipreading cues. Many video conferencing platforms provide ASR captions, although details vary by platform. While ASR captioning can be less accurate than CART, particularly with jargon, it may be sufficient for everyday and impromptu meetings.

- If you require CART, the same rules apply as for an in-person meeting.

- If the meeting is captioned, request the transcript to fill in any information you missed.

Set yourself up for listening success:
- On video calls, use speaker mode rather than gallery mode to enlarge the speaker's image, making it easier to speechread. Speaker mode also makes it easier to identify who is speaking.

- Stream to your hearing devices for the best-quality sound and to block out background noises in your location. Or use noise-cancelling headphones for the same result.

- Use assistive listening technology as needed, particularly if captioning is not available.

32

TRAVELING

WHY IS IT that anytime something goes wrong with your hearing or your hearing devices, it's when you are far away from home and from your usual sources of hearing help? People speaking with accents add another layer of complexity to your communication.

But we wouldn't miss the spectacle and magic of travel for the world. These Hearing Hacks will send you on your way with confidence.

MUST-HAVES ON EVERY TRIP

Bring extras of everything:

- Back-up hearing aids and lots of spare batteries and wax guards.

- Chargers (at least two) to keep your devices working. You may also need adaptors for other countries' electrical outlets.

- Portable drying aid for devices.

- Spare contact lenses or glasses (when you need to see to hear).

Pack your technology tools:

- Bring a *shake-awake device* (programmable vibrating pads placed under or attached to your pillow). Portable travel versions are widely available. Or use a wearable, like an Apple Watch or Fitbit.

- Use noise-cancelling headphones to prevent tinnitus spikes brought on by travel noise, especially on airplanes.

Don't forget these important items:

- The ID numbers for your devices if you need to contact the manufacturer for help.

- Your HCP's contact information.

- A travel hearing buddy! A partner, friend, or child will do for hearing help and good company.

AIR, TRAIN, AND BUS TRAVEL

Make and manage your reservations online:

- Download each carrier's app and get alerts for flight delays and gate changes sent to your smartphone. This beats trying to hear the garbled terminal announcements.

Self-identify to smooth the way:

- Disclose your hearing loss at the check-in gate, and if there are no visual indicators, ask them to alert you when it is your time to board. They may even let you board first.

- Onboard, let others, including your seatmate, know you may need assistance in an emergency or clarification of any announcements.

AT A HOTEL

Include your hearing loss in your reservation (your needs may be different if you have a travel companion):

- Follow up with the hotel and request an accessible room with an alerting light and any other accommodations you might need.

- Remind hotel staff at check-in so they know someone must retrieve you if there is an emergency during the night.

GRAND TOURS, EXCURSIONS, AND TOURIST ATTRACTIONS

Follow the tips in "Visiting a Museum or Gallery or Taking a Guided Tour" on page 243.

CAR TRAVEL

Drive with care:

- When you are the driver, find the best way to hear in the car while staying safe. Remote mics can help, especially with passengers in the back seat.

- Use a large rearview mirror to give you a better view of traffic behind you, beside you, and in your blind spot.

- Place a small extra mirror on top of the rearview mirror for a full view of the back seat passengers (particularly useful with small children).

Be prepared if stopped by the police:

- Speechreading may be tough at night, especially with a light shining in your face. Consider carrying a card that identifies your hearing loss and what you need.

- Consider a card that provides pictures of typical items like a driver's license or registration so officers can point to what they need from you.

- Keep paper and pen available for writing notes if needed.

When you are a passenger:

- Sit in the front seat. This gives you the best opportunity to speechread other passengers and the voices of those behind you will at least be aimed in your direction.

- If the incessant white noise of the road bothers you, consider wearing noise-cancelling headphones.

33

EXERCISE CLASSES

People with hearing loss may be skeptical about exercise and yoga classes. Will we be able to hear the instructor well enough to follow along in a class? Will our devices stay firmly in place or fly across the room? What about sweat?

These are real concerns, but ones that can be offset by choosing the right classes, understanding instructors, and using other Hearing Hacks.

Find the right studio or gym:

- Visit a few studios and gyms in your area to see what they offer.

- Speak to each manager about your hearing loss and how they can accommodate you.

Set yourself up for a successful class experience:

- Learn about the poses or moves in advance of classes through new-student workshops or online videos at home. This will make it easier to follow instructions during class.

- Go with a hearing buddy who is comfortable with you watching them and follow them during the class.

- Tell the instructor about your hearing loss before class. It is typical for students to discuss physical limitations with instructors before class.

- If you have a remote microphone that streams to your devices, ask the instructor to wear it.

- Location! Location! Location! Find a central spot in the room with sightlines of both the instructor and other participants in all directions.

- Use a headband to protect your devices and hold them in place.

Protect your hearing:
- Choose a class with no music or quiet music. This makes it easier to follow along with verbal commands.

- If you *must* go to a *very loud* boot camp, dance, spin class, and so on, protect your residual hearing from possible further damage by wearing ear coverings or removing your devices completely and wearing earplugs.

Try a virtual class:
- Stream a class from your computer directly to your hearing devices via Bluetooth. Choose a class with little or no music to make instructions easier to hear.

- If you prefer to use captions, try a pre-recorded class on YouTube.

- Watch a new class a few times before doing it to learn the moves. Pre-recorded videos have the added benefit of letting you pause and rewind if you miss something. Video classes are also a great way to learn new exercises before heading into a live class.

Enjoy!

- Have fun and enjoy the health benefits. Who cares if you don't get everything right the first time, or even the second?

- Don't give up if your first attempt is a dud. Try another class, instructor, or setting. It's like trying out hearing aids or frogs— the first one you kiss might not be a good match.

34

OUTDOOR ACTIVITIES

O THERWISE FUN AND healthy outdoor activities can be tricky for people with hearing loss. Imagine trying to speechread while navigating rocky terrain. Your eyes can't be in two places at once! Water sports are challenging for the simple reason that devices must not get wet. But there are strategies to make it work.

HIKING, WALKING, SNOWSHOEING, SKIING

Set ground rules ahead of time:

- Let others know that conversation may be tricky and figure out visual signals that can be used even from a distance to indicate "Let's stop" or "Shh, look over there!"

- Know the planned route in case you get separated from the group and can't hear or understand voices calling from afar.

Stay connected:

- To better hear conversations or the hike leader, position yourself to suit your listening needs.

- Take advantage of your hearing devices' directional microphones, if so equipped, by turning your head in the direction of the speaker. Bluetooth remote microphones can stream a group leader's voice into your devices.

- Encourage your companions to share the transmitter among them, when necessary, to help you hear.

CYCLING

Do all the above, plus:

- Always wear hearing devices and a helmet that fits well with them.

- Reduce wind noise in hearing aids with headbands or noise reducers designed for helmets.

- Use rearview mirrors on both handlebars to stay alert to traffic all around you.

BOATING AND OTHER WATER ACTIVITIES

Develop communications guidelines:

- The sound of the waves and the wind in your ears can be noisy. Warn others that communication may be tough, especially if you must remove your devices to keep them safe and dry.

- Adopt some simple signs, like those used by scuba divers or some of your own design, to communicate at distances across the water.

- Appoint a hearing buddy who can help you understand the instructions from emergency personnel or other speakers.

Plan for your devices:
- If you leave them at home, they are safe—but you may not be able to converse.

- Consider using old devices instead, if you have ones that work well enough to provide some sound.

- If you can't do without your regular devices, when not in use, store them with their cases in a drybag or a waterproof case, or even in a heavy-duty plastic zip bag. Most dry bags can be clipped to the boat to prevent your devices from going overboard.

- Bring an emergency drying aid in case your devices get soaked. Small travel drying aids are available for a low price, or you can make your own with a sachet of silica gel or rice.

- Wear a headband or sport band to keep your hearing aids and sound processors in place.

Always do this after-care:

- Inspect the devices for sand and debris and remove any with a damp cloth.

- Once off the water, use a hair dryer on a cool setting to dry out wet devices. Hold them at least a couple feet from the dryer.

- If anything sounds odd the next day, take your hearing aids to your HCP as soon as possible.

THE JOURNEY CONTINUES

A ND—THAT'S A WRAP! Everything we know about the hearing loss journey, offered in the simplest way we know how!

We illuminated the Big Picture—the typical hearing loss journey comprising five stages. We perched on our favorite three-legged stool of strategies—MindShifts, Technology, and Communication Game Changers. We expanded our focus from hearing better to communicating better. And on almost every page, we examined the impact of hearing loss on our lives—how our emotions and attitudes can change the way we interact with others.

Hearing loss is universal in scope, yet intensely personal. We hope you have recognized at least some parts of your life on these pages.

Use *Hear & Beyond* as a valuable reference, to revisit whenever you need ideas and support. We hope it inspires a renewed commitment to live skillfully with your hearing loss and helps you find the confidence to move forward. Sharing it with the people in your life will help them better understand what you need from them.

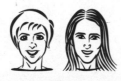

Living skillfully with hearing loss is an ongoing process, and so, for each of us, the journey continues.

We encourage you to keep learning about hearing loss. Read articles and books—and read this one again! There are also many superb informational websites and social media outlets that can help you solve problems and create your path forward. Or sit down with your trusted hearing care professional to discuss the tough questions. And if you haven't done so already, reach out to others who have hearing loss—to share experiences and to learn from each other. It's life-changing—that's a promise.

Finally, we invite you to connect with us. Contact us through our social media platforms, our blogs, or our book's website. We would love to hear from you.

HearAndBeyond.com
ShariEberts.com
GaelHannan.com

Living skillfully with hearing loss is an ongoing process, and so, for each of us, the journey continues.

ACKNOWLEDGMENTS

H*ear & Beyond* has been a labor of love, and one that rests on the shoulders of many thought leaders, advocates, and hearing loss friends. We are grateful for the knowledge and inspiration we found in the research, writing, and work of many in the industry including Charles Laszlo, Marshall Chasin, Joanne DeLuzio, Glynnis Tidball, and Ida Institute for their work promoting person-centered hearing care. We also thank Ida Institute, *The Hearing Journal*, and *Hearing Health & Technology Matters* for allowing us to adapt and include some material that we originally wrote for them.

We are indebted to our fellow advocates—there are too many to name—as well as consumer organizations like the Canadian Hard of Hearing Association and Hearing Loss Association of America that work tirelessly on behalf of people with hearing loss to raise awareness and provide education and support.

Thank you to our early readers Holly Cohen, Cindy Gordon, Richard Einhorn, Kevin Liebe, Barbara Weinstein, and Joanne DeLuzio, and to Wayne Lilley for his early editing. You each confirmed for us that we were on the right path, and your suggestions, refinements, and redirects helped us to make this the best book we could. Thanks also to our husbands for their perceptive insights into the topics we should cover and the best way to express our ideas.

Thank you to our hearing loss friends around the world. We feel your support, love, and encouragement every day of our lives. You inspire us to advocate for ourselves and others and you pick us up when we grow weary. A special callout to our fellow Victorious women Holly Cohen, Peggy Ellertsen, Cindy Gordon, Toni Iacolucci, and Roxana Rotundo. Your friendship means the world to us.

We are grateful for the professional stewardship of our publishing team at Page Two. Thank you to Jesse Finkelstein for recognizing the need for *Hear & Beyond* and for pushing us to make it the valuable reference tool we hope it has become. Special thanks to our incredible editor, Kendra Ward, and copy editor, Rachel Ironstone, who helped us shape our baby into its current form, and to our marketer extraordinaire, Chris Brandt.

Thank you to our families for their love and support every day and in every way: Ken, Aerin, and Alden Eberts and the Hannans—Doug (the Hearing Husband), Joel, Jacqui, Katie, Chris, Morgan, Scott, Kristina, and all the little ones. We love you.

And last but not least, a special thank you to each other. As two fiercely independent writers, we learned to trust the process, even when things got jiggly. We believe in each other and the power of collaboration, and what we created together reflects who we are as individuals and our shared philosophies. We are proud to share it with the world.

NOTES

1. Wikipedia, s.v. "Most Common Words in English," accessed April 21, 2021, en.wikipedia.org/wiki/Most_common_words_in_English.

2. "Diabetes and Hearing Loss," American Diabetes Association, accessed June 21, 2021, diabetes.org/diabetes-and-hearing-loss; David R. Friedland, Christopher Cederberg, and Sergey Tarima, "Audiometric Pattern as a Predictor of Cardiovascular Status: Development of a Model for Assessment of Risk," *The Laryngoscope* 119, no. 3 (February 2009): 473–86, doi.org/10.1002/lary.20130.

3. Johns Hopkins Medicine, "Hearing Loss Linked to Three-fold Risk of Falling," News and Publications, release date February 27, 2012, hopkinsmedicine.org/news/media/releases/hearing_loss_linked_to_three_fold_risk_of_falling.

4. Johns Hopkins Medicine, "Hearing Loss and Dementia Linked in Study," News and Publications, release date February 14, 2011, hopkinsmedicine.org/news/media/releases/hearing_loss_and_dementia_linked_in_study.

5. Hélène Amevia, Camille Ouvrard, Caroline Giulioli, Céline Meillon, Laetitia Rullier, and Jean-François Dartigues, "Self-Reported Hearing Loss, Hearing Aids, and Cognitive Decline in Elderly Adults: A 25-Year Study," *Journal of the American Geriatrics Society* 63, no. 10 (October 2015): 2099–104, doi.org/10.1111/jgs.13649; Gill Livingston, Jonathan Huntley, Andrew Sommerlad, David Ames, Clive Ballard, Sube Banerjee, Carol Brayne, et al., "Dementia Prevention, Intervention, and Care: 2020 Report of the *Lancet* Commission," *The Lancet Commissions* 396, no. 10248 (August 2020): 413–46, doi.org/10.1016/S0140-6736(20)30367-6.

6. "All About Tinnitus," British Tinnitus Association, accessed June 21, 2021, tinnitus.org.uk/all-about-tinnitus.

7. "WHO: 1 in 4 People Projected to Have Hearing Problems by 2050," World Health Organization, March 2, 2021, who.int/news/item/02-03-2021-who-1-in-4-people-projected-to-have-hearing-problems-by-2050.

8. For example, see Christopher N. Cascio, Matthew Brook O'Donnell, Francis J. Tinney, Matthew D. Lieberman, Shelley E. Taylor, Victor J. Stretcher, and Emily B. Falk, "Self-affirmation Activates Brain Systems Associated with Self-related Processing and Reward and Is Reinforced by Future Orientation," *Social Cognitive and Affective Neuroscience* 11, no. 4 (April 2016): 621–29, doi.org/10.1093/scan/nsv136.

9. Carol L. Flinchbaugh, E. Whitney G. Moore, Young K. Chang, and Douglas R. May, "Student Well-being Interventions: The Effects of Stress Management Techniques and Gratitude Journaling in the Management Education Classroom," *Journal of Management Education* 36, no. 2 (April 2012): 191–219, doi.org/10.1177/1052562911430062; Leah Dickens and David DeSteno, "The Grateful Are Patient: Heightened Daily Gratitude Is Associated with Attenuated Temporal Discounting," *Emotion* 16, no. 4 (2016): 421–25, doi.org/10.1037/emo0000176; Alex M. Wood, Stephen Joseph, Joanna Lloyd, and Samuel Atkins, "Gratitude Influences Sleep through the Mechanism of Pre-sleep Cognitions," *Journal of Psychosomatic Research* 66, no. 1 (January 2009): 43–48, doi.org/10.1016/j.jpsychores.2008.09.002; Prathik Kini, Joel Wong, Sydney McInnis, Nicole Gabana, and Joshua W. Brown, "The Effects of Gratitude Expression on Neural Activity," *NeuroImage* 128 (March 2016): 1–10, doi.org/10.1016/j.neuroimage.2015.12.040.

10. John Geraci, *AARP/American Speech-Language-Hearing Association (ASHA): National Poll on Hearing Health Results Summary* (New York: Crux Research, Inc., 2011).

11. "Too Loud. Too Long." It's a Noisy Planet, accessed June 21, 2021, noisyplanet.nidcd.nih.gov/parents/too-loud-too-long.

12. Brennan R. Payne, Jack W. Silcox, Hannah A. Crandell, Amanda Lash, Sarah Hargus Ferguson, and Monika Lohani, "Text Captioning Buffers Against the Effects of Background Noise and Hearing Loss on Memory for Speech," *Ear and Hearing* (July 12, 2021): doi.org/10.1097/AUD.0000000000001079; S. Adam Brasel and James Gips, "Enhancing Television Advertising: Same-Language Subtitles Can Improve Brand Recall, Verbal Memory, and Behavioral Intent," *Journal of the Academy of Marketing Science* 42, no. 3 (May 2014): 322–36, doi.org/10.1007/s11747-013-0358-1.

13. The sample communication access plan can be accessed at hearingloss.org/wp-content/uploads/HLAA_HC_Full_Guide.pdf or by simply googling "HLAA communication access plan."

INDEX

SHARI EBERTS is a passionate hearing health advocate and internationally recognized author and speaker on hearing loss issues. She founded LivingWithHearingLoss.com, a popular blog and online community for people living with hearing loss and tinnitus, and is an executive producer of *We Hear You*, an award-winning documentary about the hearing loss experience. Shari also serves on the board of directors of Hearing Loss Association of America.

Shari has an adult-onset genetic hearing loss and hopes that by sharing her story she will help others to live more peacefully with their own hearing issues. Her writing has been featured in the *Washington Post*, *Psychology Today*, *Huffington Post*, *Good Housekeeping*, *Woman's Day*, *The Hearing Journal*, and numerous other publications. Shari is also the editor of FindHearing for *Hearing Health & Technology Matters*.

Prior to her advocacy work, Shari had a twenty-year career in finance. She holds a BS in Psychology summa cum laude from Duke University and an MBA from Harvard Business School. She lives in New York City with her husband and two children.

Connect with Shari on her website ShariEberts.com or on Twitter @sharieberts.